Ageless Attitude

Enlightened, Empowered and Excited:
A Practical Guide to Effortless Ageing

Stu and Sue Roberts

Ageless Attitude

Enlightened, Empowered and Excited: A Practical Guide to Effortless Ageing

© 2025 Cobb Alexander Limited

All rights reserved.

No part of this publication may be reproduced, stored in a retrieval system, or transmitted in any form or by any means (electronic, mechanical, photocopying, recording, scanning or otherwise) without the prior written permission of the publisher, except in the case of brief quotations used in reviews or articles.

ISBN: 9781068188800 (Paperback)

Published by: Inspired By Publishing

Disclaimer

This book is intended for informational and inspirational purposes only. It reflects the authors' personal insights, research, and experiences in exploring mindset and ageing. It is not intended to provide professional medical, health, or psychological advice, diagnosis or treatment. It should not be used as a substitute for consultation with qualified health or wellness professionals.

Readers are encouraged to take full responsibility for their own choices and wellbeing, and to consult qualified professionals regarding their health, wellness or ageing-related concerns.

The ideas, strategies, insights, and suggestions in this book are based on the authors' personal experiences and research and are offered in good faith. The author and publisher make no representations or warranties as to the completeness or accuracy of the content, nor do they accept any liability for any loss, injury, or damage allegedly arising from the use or application of the information contained in this book. Every effort has been made to trace copyright holders and obtain permission for the use of third-party material.

There is no guarantee that readers will achieve the same outcomes or experiences as the authors. Individual results may vary, and applying the guidance in this book is at the reader's own discretion and risk.

The authors reserve the right to make changes to the content at any time and assume no responsibility or liability whatsoever on behalf of any purchaser or reader of these materials.

For our parents.

If the knowledge now available on ageing well had been more widely known in your time, your final chapter might have been very different. May this book honour your legacy in some small way and offer a hopeful guide to those seeking to embrace ageing with empowered possibility.

Acknowledgements

As with any passion project, there are so many people we want to thank for their invaluable contributions and support.

To list them down chronologically, we'd like to start with our amazing mentors. We've been incredibly fortunate to have learned from them via coaching, courses and books. The power of mindset was first introduced to us by Peter Thomson. His engaging and inspiring yet down-to-earth style was a revelation for us. He introduced us to a world of personal development that previously we'd been put off by, as in those days, it did have a bit of a worthy "hessian-weave" vibe. Peter introduced us to the work of Deepak Chopra, who, along with Dr. Michael Colgan, Dr. Lawrence Plaskett and Joe Dispenza, opened our eyes to the body's amazing capacity to keep fit and healthy as we age.

More recently, Patrick Holford has been an inspiration to us on how to age well. Paul O'Mahoney, Peter Sage, Robin Banks and Yvette Wearne have been instrumental in helping us harness the power of our minds and apply our learning to our approach to ageing.

To our insightful and intuitive coaches, Isabelle Moreau and Shereen Malika, we can't thank you enough for supporting us through the challenging times that catalysed the writing of this book.

The brilliant team at Inspired By Publishing have been amazing; thank you. Attending Chloë Bisson's Writing Challenge was truly inspirational and provided a comprehensive toolkit to translate the vague embryo of an idea into a tangible manuscript. Huge thanks to our writing mentor, Zena Search, who patiently kept us focused on structuring our ideas. Then in the Editorial and Ops Teams, Alex, Lottie, Kat, Camyl and Mia – your energy, drive and legendary eye for detail have been amazing. We are incredibly grateful for your support and for always being so motivating in transforming our typed documents into a book.

Finally, our beloved family supported us with unconditional love and a sense of fun throughout this whole venture. We can't thank them enough for being fabulous and unwitting barometers for how to address certain subjects. Their glazed expressions and the silent rolling of eyes were great indicators for editing ideas that may not be quite so interesting to others as they were to us! You have contributed far more than you'll ever know!

Foreword

I think there comes a time in all our lives when we are called to pause, reflect and re-evaluate everything we thought we knew. For Stu and Sue Roberts, that moment arrived with the passing of their ageing parents.

This was a season defined by deep grief, but also by extraordinary clarity. In the face of their deep loss, a deeper truth emerged: that how we age and how we approach ageing in those we love matters profoundly. This book is a beautiful and powerful response to the truth that was born from these very sad yet defining moments for Stu and Sue.

This book is not a manual on how to reverse ageing, nor is it an attempt to deny the natural changes that come with time. The book shares from a space of deep compassion and care and it is an empowering invitation to reframe our relationship with ageing itself. It asks us to challenge the outdated belief that getting older means becoming less. And instead, it offers a bold, uplifting alternative, that ageing can be a journey of expansion, wisdom, vitality and even joy.

When I had the privilege of working with Stu and Sue during the Mind Power Course, I was struck by their dedication to personal growth, their courage to question convention and their clarity of purpose. I saw two people fully committed to living intentionally and equally committed to guiding others to do the same. This is all exemplified by the love they not only share for each other but for humanity.

What they've created here is a deeply honest and hopeful book. It offers practical tools grounded in science, profound insights rooted in personal experience and a fresh, enlightened perspective on what it means to age well. It blends heart and mind in a way that feels both intimate and universal, as well as exciting!

The book is a reminder that we are always "becoming." That each chapter of our lives, regardless of our age, can be lived fully, joyfully and with deep meaning.

To Stu and Sue, I am honoured to have played a part in your journey and proud to see the incredible work you've brought into the world. I am excited to share the rest with you and witness the profound teachings, sharing and transformation that this next chapter holds not only for you but for us as a planet.

To the very special human who reads this book, my wish for you is that this book challenges you, uplifts you and reminds you that it's never too late to live with purpose, passion and power.

Yours in love and light,

Yvette Wearne
Lead Mind Power Coach and Manager
International Team of Coaches
Robin Banks & Associates

Contents

Introduction	1
Chapter 1 - Our Perception of Ageing	9
Chapter 2 - Mind-Body Connection	29
Chapter 3 - Life Wisdom	73
Chapter 4 - Know Thyself	93
Chapter 5 - Navigating Life's Challenges	113
Chapter 6 - Purpose and Passion	147
Chapter 7 - Nothing Is Learned Until It Is Lived	167
Chapter 8 - Keeping a Sense of Wonder	187
Conclusion: Ageing as a Journey of Empowerment	213
Further Resources	219
References	223
Bibliography	229

Introduction

"The greatest discovery of any generation is that a human being can alter his life by altering his attitude."

– William James

Hello!

If you've picked up this book, chances are you're curious about ageing. Maybe you're approaching what society calls "later life" and wondering what's ahead. Maybe you've watched loved ones struggle through their older years, as we have, and you're searching for a way to approach this inevitable chapter of life with hope rather than dread. Or maybe you're simply someone who believes, deep down, that there's a better way to think about growing older – one that doesn't involve fear, resignation or a desperate scramble for the latest anti-ageing gimmick. As co-authors of this book, we, Stu and Sue, believe there is, and we're excited to share that vision with you.

Ageing doesn't have to be a story of decline. It doesn't have to be a battle against time or a grim march toward frailty and irrelevance. Ageing, as the inimitable David Bowie once said, "is an extraordinary process where you become the person you always should have been." What if, instead of fearing this process, we embraced it as an opportunity to step into our fullest, wisest, most vibrant selves? What if we could shift our perspective to see ageing not as a loss, but as a gain? A chance to live with greater purpose, passion and joy?

This book is about empowering you to do just that. It's not about nutrition plans, exercise regimes, or supplements. There are plenty of excellent resources out there for those. Instead, this book dives into something far more personal and, we believe, far more powerful: the role our thoughts, emotions and outlook play in how we age. While we can't control everything about our health in later life, we can control how we think, how we feel and how we choose to see the world. And those choices, as you'll discover, have a profound impact on our wellbeing – physically, mentally and emotionally.

The Catalyst for This Book

After months of COVID lockdowns preventing us from visiting Stu's mum, we were finally granted permission to see her in the hospital in the last week of her life. Some people say that you should not see a loved one before they die if they are in a bad way, as that image gets chiselled into your mind. It becomes your defining recollection of them, overshadowing all other memories for what feels like an age. Others say it's vital to be there, even if they're unconscious, so you can say goodbye. Whatever you choose, it feels like there's no right answer. Stu was still questioning his decision even as we followed the duty nurse to his mum's room. The corridor seemed endless, dimly lit and cloaked in that sterile, chemical, distinctive hospital smell. The walls, a lifeless shade of grey, closed in around us with every step.

Our legs felt heavy, as though we were wading through concrete, each footstep bringing us closer to something we didn't want to face. As the nurse opened the door, her expression should have warned us. But nothing could have prepared us for what we found.

The woman we knew – vibrant, always beautifully dressed and perfectly blow-dried hair, justly proud of her slim, dancer's physique – was not the person lying in that hospital bed. Instead of the woman we knew, there was a tiny, emaciated figure, her once beautiful hair gone, every breath a loud, reverberating, rasping struggle that echoed hauntingly along the corridor. In Stu's 30 years as an operational firefighter, he had seen some harrowing sights. But nothing had left him feeling this shocked. Holding her brittle hand, we both told her how much we loved her and thanked her for all the fun times we had shared together. Stu whispered that it was time for her to let go, but the emotional weight was so overwhelming that he could only stay a few more minutes before leaving, unable to return.

Sixteen years earlier, we had watched helplessly when Stu's dad had endured a painful death in the hospital. All the memories of that excruciating time came flooding back.

It was a similarly heartbreaking experience with Sue's dad in 2015. Like Stu's mum, this was someone who had always been physically fit; running upstairs, leapfrogging over bollards on his way to the train station, a man we never saw as "old." So, it was a cannonball blow to the stomach when we learned he had just months to live following a small-cell lung cancer diagnosis. Watching helplessly as his health deteriorated at lightning speed, we couldn't fathom how, just a short time before, he'd been so full

INTRODUCTION

of life. That interminable last night in the hospital, as he slipped away at just 76, left a massive gap in our family's life.

Within a month or so of Stu's mum's death, Sue's mum's health declined significantly. She had had ongoing issues from sepsis a few years previously, and now was evidently suffering from dementia. This most caring and thoughtful of people, so full of love and always there to help others, was now needing to be the person being helped – a complete anathema for her. Being so self-reliant and independent, it was devastating for her devoted family to make the tough decision that to keep her safe, she needed to live in the gilded cage of a care home. Again, not the final chapter we would have wanted for this treasured mum, mother-in-law and adored grandmother.

Your life can feel like it's on hold, weighed down by responsibility and grief. There's a constant nagging feeling of guilt, wondering if you've made the right decisions for their care and wondering if you've done enough. It's easy to lose hope and momentum for your own future.

Like many of our friends facing similar challenges, a question often arises, *"Will this be me in 20 or 30 years?"* It can feel selfish asking yourself this, but it's also practical and caring, as you don't want your children or nieces and nephews to endure the distress and pressure that you have.

Mortified that we were not able to protect our parents from these traumatic last chapters of their lives, we were ignited with a determination to support others facing similar heartache and to find ways to help people build a strong foundation for their own long-term health. Death is inevitable, but the extent to which we suffer before our departure is not.

We were keen to turn our experience into something positive. This book came from our quest to find a different way forward. You don't need to have supported ill parents for this book to be relevant to you. If there's a part of you that is starting to wonder what your older years will bring, then you're in the right place too.

We've immersed ourselves in research, absorbing knowledge from books, studies and what feels like continuous courses! This book is here to share what we have learned from all this research, as well as the insights and experience we have gained through trial and error. If you currently feel fearful or resigned, our hope is that you'll feel optimistic, inspired and ready to embrace your later years of life with clarity, purpose and enthusiasm.

Health in later life is, of course, shaped by a complex web of factors, many of which can feel out of our control. One area where we have immense power is in our thoughts, emotions and outlook on life. The more we explored this, the more we realised how transformative it can be. Our thoughts and emotions aren't just fleeting reactions; they're powerful forces that can literally change our biology, shape our resilience and determine how we age.

What This Book Is and Isn't

This book is not, of course, a promise of eternal youth or a denial of the realities of ageing. We all get older. Our bodies change.

INTRODUCTION

Challenges arise. But this book is about reframing those realities, about challenging the outdated narrative that ageing is something to fear or fight. It's about giving you the tools to approach this chapter of life with optimism, wisdom and resilience.

Here's what you can expect as you turn these pages. We'll start by examining how our perception of ageing is shaped – by society, by media, by the stories we've been told – and how we can challenge that old paradigm to create a new, more empowering one (Chapter 1). From there, we'll explore the mind-body connection, revealing the extraordinary power your thoughts and emotions have over your biochemistry (Chapter 2).

We both reached 60 and didn't feel that we were the wise people we'd expected ourselves to be by the time we reached our 7th decade! So, if you're feeling similar to the way we were then, Chapter 3 will help to remind you of the knowledge and experience you've accumulated over the years and turn it into a source of strength and vitality. And if you're already feeling like a Wise Elder, this chapter will help you tap further into your incredible reservoir of wisdom.

In Chapter 4, "Know Thyself," we'll reflect on David Bowie's words and explore the importance of tuning into your unique needs and being true to who you are. This chapter also introduces the concept of bio-individuality, as there's no one-size-fits-all approach to ageing well.

Chapter 5, "Navigating Life's Challenges," will offer practical ways to face the inevitable difficulties of later life – whether it's bereavement, caring for elderly parents or managing health issues – with grace and resourcefulness.

Being true to ourselves and having a clear direction are important throughout life. In Chapter 6, "Purpose & Passion," we'll explore its significance as we get older and the role it plays in longevity. We have both been guilty of reading books and attending courses, feeling fired up by the knowledge and insights, then not actually applying our learning. So, in Chapter 7, "Nothing Is Learned Until It Is Lived," we provide practical ways for you to integrate your valuable experience and the new information you've acquired into your life. And finally, in Chapter 8, "Sense of Wonder," we'll rediscover the childlike curiosity and awe that helps us find the extraordinary in the ordinary. And while "wonder" might sound whimsical, research suggests it can do wonders, quite literally, for our long-term wellbeing.

Why This Matters

We believe that how we age is one of the most important conversations we can have, not just for ourselves, but for our families, our communities and the generations that follow. The way we approach ageing shapes not only our own lives but also the cultural narrative about what it means to grow older. And there's never been a more urgent time to have this conversation. With an ageing global population, increasing awareness of mental and emotional wellbeing and a growing desire to live not just longer but better, now is the moment to take charge of how you age. Now is the time to rewrite the story before challenges arise, to build resilience before it's tested and to embrace ageing as a journey of growth, not decline. By embracing ageing with optimism, we can inspire others to do the same, creating a ripple effect of hope and empowerment.

INTRODUCTION

As you read this book, we invite you to approach it with an open mind and a willing heart. Some of the ideas may challenge long-held beliefs. Others may feel like a warm confirmation of what you've always known deep down. Either way, our hope is that these pages will inspire you, equip you to find what works for you, and remind you that ageing is not something to endure, but something to embrace – a journey of becoming, of unfolding, of stepping into the truest expression of who you are so you can live your life to the full.

So, let's get started.

CHAPTER 1
Our Perception of Ageing

Harry: Do you ever think about death?

Sally: Yes.

Harry: Sure you do, a fleeting thought that jumps in and out of the transient of your mind. I spend hours, I spend days...

Sally: And you think that makes you a better person.

Harry: Look, when the shit comes down, I'm gonna be prepared and you're not. That's all I'm saying.

Sally: And in the meantime, you're gonna ruin your whole life waiting for it.

– Nora Ephron, *When Harry Met Sally* (film script)

OUR PERCEPTION OF AGEING

At what point do you consider someone to be "old"?

Is it when they reach a particular birthday? When their hair turns grey? When their body starts to slow down? Or is it something less tangible, like a shift in attitude, energy or outlook? When you notice they frequently moan about the current state of the world and compare it unfavourably with the past. Maybe it's when they stop being curious about new ideas, resist change or become more rigid in their thinking. That subtle narrowing of perspective, the loss of openness, humour or vitality, can sometimes make someone seem "old" regardless of their actual age.

Ask five people the same question and you'll get five different responses. How we answer this question is deeply personal, shaped by a lifetime of influences: family experiences, media messages, cultural norms and the roles we see older people playing in society. Many of these beliefs live just below the surface, quietly colouring how we see ourselves as we grow older.

So why does this matter?

Because the way we perceive ageing has a big impact on the way we age: our energy, our self-esteem, our relationships, even our health. If we carry around outdated ideas that growing older means decline, limitation or being less relevant, we're more likely to live as if that were true. We may slow ourselves down unnecessarily, hold ourselves back, shrink our ambitions or feel like our best years are behind us, even when they're not. We may feel less confident, less visible or even fear becoming a burden.

That's the real risk: not ageing itself, but what we miss out on when we believe the old story.

In lots of the traditional support for approaching ageing, there's often an underlying theme that ageing is about coping. Surface-level strategies tend to be covered: dealing with declining physical health, financial planning and preparing for retirement. And while these are important, they don't tell the whole story. What's often missing is the inner work: how our thoughts, feelings and beliefs profoundly shape how we age. That's what we're going to focus on.

As mentioned in the introduction, rather than fixating on what's beyond your control, we focus on what *is* within your reach: your mindset, your emotions, your outlook. We'll explore the powerful connection between mind and body, the value of life wisdom, the importance of staying curious and the vital role of purpose and passion. You'll be invited to savour each day, reconnect with what lights you up and apply what you learn. This is so ageing becomes something to grow into, not something to resist or fear. You don't have to follow the old version of what ageing means. You get to define it yourself.

Thankfully, when we do let go of the old paradigm and embrace a new perception of ageing, something powerful happens. We start to notice possibilities instead of limitations. We feel more vital, more present, more open to new experiences. We stop judging ourselves by how many candles are on our birthday cake and start focusing on what truly matters: how we feel, how we live and how connected we are to our purpose, our passions and to the people we care about. Changing how we *see* ageing is the first step to changing how we *experience* it.

Recent research in the fields of psychology, neuroscience and gerontology supports this: Our beliefs about ageing can significantly influence our physical health, cognitive function and even longevity. A Yale University study in 2002 was the first to show that people with a more positive view of ageing live, on average, 7.5 years longer than those with negative age beliefs.[1] Our mindset affects our biology. It can impact stress levels, resilience and even how well we recover from illness. In short, changing how we think about ageing isn't just uplifting; it's life-enhancing.

In this chapter, we'll explore the many sources, both overt and subtle, that shape our current outlook. So many of our thoughts and feelings about ageing are absorbed unconsciously throughout our lives. These thoughts and feelings are effectively second-hand opinions. This chapter gives you the chance to review your own perceptions so that you can decide, with greater clarity, which ones to keep and which to let go of.

How Ageing Can Take Us by Surprise

Accepting that we're in our latter years comes as a surprise to most of us. The realisation hits us all at different times. For some, it's that first zero birthday when you realise you're more than halfway through your life. Perhaps when you reached your 50th birthday, it felt okay, as there's a chance of living to 100, but maybe when you turned 60, it felt like a whole different ball game. Sometimes it's that first funeral of a parent, aunt or uncle that triggers the thought that you're the next generation in line on that conveyor belt of life. In terms of day-to-day practicalities, being entitled to discounted cinema tickets or cheaper rail fares provides evidence of being considered old. Ticking the age range box in online questionnaires and needing to scroll down much closer to the bottom of the list is also a reminder of the number of years that have gone by and how few date ranges are left to choose from! Do any of these resonate with you? What were your first realisations?

Common Fears About Ageing

Ageing was traditionally seen as the autumn and winter of our lives, a stage of loss and decline. Over the last few decades, there has been a significant shift based on cultural, scientific and social changes. So ageing is evolving to be embraced as a period of wisdom, growth and self-fulfilment.

Despite this paradigm change, as with any big transformation, it's more oil tanker than speedboat in altering course. Through the millennia of human evolution, in order to survive, we developed an inbuilt protection system for prioritising fear-based thoughts. This is so hard-wired in our brains that it takes conscious effort to recognise the negative bias. "The 5-to-1 Rule" indicates that it takes around five positive thoughts to outweigh the impact of a single negative one. So, when we might feel a sense of dread or worry about what's to come, we need to remind ourselves to counteract it with five positive perceptions. Being aware of this default programming helps to observe more objectively some of the fears that many of us have assimilated about ageing. Surveys and research studies on the fear of ageing cite a wide array of people's concerns. Which of these common fears resonate with you?

☐ Declining physical health

☐ Declining mental health

☐ Loss of mobility

☐ Losing independence

- ☐ Loss of identity or sense of purpose

- ☐ Lack of relevance in youth-oriented cultures

- ☐ Being a burden to loved ones

- ☐ Death and what happens after

- ☐ Social isolation

- ☐ Loss of youthful physical appearance

- ☐ Loss of dignity

- ☐ Not achieving personal dreams and goals

Messages We Absorb About Ageing

It is fascinating how ageing is viewed by different cultures and societies around the world, and the corresponding impact this conditioning can have on our outlook. We are surrounded by information that promotes this negative perspective of getting old.

Family. If your grandparents lived to 100, smoked 60 cigarettes a day, were full of vigour and died peacefully in their sleep, you'll probably have a different perception from someone who witnessed frail grandparents losing their independence and dying in pain in hospital after a long illness.

Language. Studies have shown that the language we use for youth is far more positive than the words we use to describe older people. We would describe a young person as "ambitious and full of potential." Yet the equivalent descriptor for older people with ambition is often something like "having a midlife crisis"! At what point in life should we stop being ambitious or denied the opportunity to realise our potential?!

Phrases such as "over the hill" or "past one's prime" both imply it's too late. And what about the "late bloomers", people like the famous artist, Anna Mary Robertson Moses? Known as "Grandma Moses," she had worked on a farm most of her life, and so wasn't able to dedicate time to her painting until her late seventies.

Talking about our age. Five-year-olds are very proud to say that they are 5 and a half or 5 and three-quarters, as those extra months show how grown-up they are; it's a badge of honour. Many adults are less comfortable talking about their age in professional settings or with new people. Is this because they feel they will be judged or stereotyped? It's seen as rude to ask someone how old they are. There's a subliminal message here that age is a taboo or sensitive subject. It reinforces the idea that age is something to hide, something that diminishes our value.

News, media and adverts. The news and media emphasise problems to grab our attention, which primes our minds to expect the worst or to focus on the negative. The media is full of stories of the ageing population and how society will not be able to cope with so many old people in hospitals and nursing homes in the years to come. Many adverts targeted at older people are focused on a decline in mobility, such as stairlifts, tilting chairs and walk-in baths.

Popular songs. Many songs imply a sense of regret for the passing years. Singing along to these songs indoctrinates a perception that our worth somehow diminishes with age. For example, "When I'm 64?" by The Beatles questions whether somebody will still be needed at that age. "Young and Beautiful" by Lana Del

Rey asks, "Will you still love me when I'm no longer young and beautiful?" implying that beauty and desirability fade with age.

How we age is based on our genes. It was once widely believed that our genes alone determined how we'd age and what illnesses we might eventually face. If dementia, heart disease or arthritis "ran in the family," the assumption was that we'd probably end up with them too.

But science has shown that our genes are *not* the whole story. In fact, how we live – our daily habits, emotional wellbeing, environment and even mindset can all influence which genes are "switched on" and which remain dormant. Lifestyle choices play a much bigger role in how we age than we ever imagined. And yet, many people still carry the belief that ageing is out of their hands, a biological fate written in their DNA. This can lead to two disempowering responses: either *fearing* the ageing process or *giving up*, thinking there's no point trying to improve things if the outcome is already decided. Is it any wonder, then, that many of us feel uneasy or even down about the prospect of getting older? The social messages we receive are often pessimistic, reinforcing the idea that ageing is a slow decline we can't do anything about.

Retirement Age

The concept of "retirement age" is a relatively modern invention, one that can unconsciously limit our sense of purpose and vitality. In his book Ageless Body, Timeless Mind, Deepak Chopra highlights a striking statistic: The average American dies within seven years of retirement. In some studies of early retirement, the mortality rate was even higher, leading to what some have called the "early retirement death." When society tells us that our productive years end at 60 or 65, it sends a powerful message: Your contribution is no longer valued. This can trigger a psychological shift, a quiet withdrawal from life itself. Without purpose, structure and a sense of belonging, our physical and mental health can quickly decline. But retirement doesn't have to mean retreat. In fact, it can be a doorway to reinvention; a time to explore passions, share wisdom, deepen relationships and contribute in new and fulfilling ways.

Objectively Reviewing Our Unique Perception

Of course, ageing isn't a one-size-fits-all or static concept; our perception changes throughout our lives and is influenced by a diverse range of internal and external factors. Some influences we are consciously aware of, others less so. Knowing what ageing means to us is important as it determines our approach to life. Taking the time to observe objectively our unique outlook on ageing enables us to select which thoughts and beliefs we want to keep and which ones we want to replace.

Rather like the radio chatting away in the background, it's not possible to control what is being said. However, actively choosing which station to select and which programmes to listen to helps to focus attention on what is important to you.

The more empowering the picture we have of getting older, the more inspired we'll be for the years ahead, so thoughts need to be chosen wisely. Thankfully, they are just thoughts, and thoughts can be changed. That said, some of our thoughts and beliefs are hard-wired and may take some time to be replaced.

Changing our Personal Perception of Ageing

"The curious paradox is that when I accept myself just as I am, then I can change."

– Carl Rogers

Take a few quiet moments to reflect on the following prompts. It's not about getting the "right" answers. Just allow your thoughts and ideas to flow.

- What messages about ageing did you absorb growing up: from family, films, books, media or community?

- How do these messages influence the way you feel about getting older?

- Which perceptions or assumptions no longer feel true or helpful?

- What inspiring examples (people you know or public figures) challenge those outdated beliefs?

- If you could rewrite the story of ageing for yourself, what would it sound like?

You might like to write your reflections in a journal or voice-note them for later. Often, it's in the space between awareness and intention that the most powerful transformation begins. Perception is not fixed. It is shaped by repetition, emotion and choice. In the Further Resources section at the end of this book, you'll find how to access the Companion Guide that includes exercises to explore this further.

Chronological, Biological and Psychological Age

Age isn't just about how many candles are on your birthday cake. It can be understood through three different lenses: *chronological*, *biological* and *psychological*. Each gives us a different picture of how we're ageing.

Chronological age is simply the number of years we've been alive. It's fixed and unchangeable. But that number alone doesn't define who you are or what you're capable of. A former colleague of Stu's once said, "I've stopped running to work now that I'm 50!" As if reaching that number somehow meant his body had received an expiry notice. In reality, it's not the number that slows us down; it's our belief about what that number means.

Biological age refers to how well (or not) your body is functioning, regardless of your actual age in years. It's influenced by many factors: lifestyle, diet, exercise, sleep, stress and even your mindset. Someone who eats well, moves regularly, sleeps soundly and manages stress effectively may have the heart, lungs and cells of someone 10 or 20 years younger than their chronological age. For example, 81-year-old Ernestine Shepherd – recognised as the world's oldest competitive female bodybuilder – didn't even start working out until her mid-fifties. Her biological age is likely to be far younger than her years suggest.

Psychological age is how old you *feel* and think you are. It's shaped by your outlook, emotional health, mental agility, curiosity, playfulness and sense of purpose. You've probably met someone in their thirties who seems world-weary and "old," and someone in their eighties who radiates energy, humour and enthusiasm for life. Dame Judi Dench once said, "I don't want to be told I'm too old to try something." That's psychological youth in action!

So, while we can't change our chronological age, we *can* influence both our biological and psychological age. In doing so, we can completely change our experience of growing older. This book is all about helping you do exactly that. We want to shift the focus away from defining yourself based on your chronological age and towards empowering your mind and body so they feel younger, stronger and more vibrant, no matter how many birthdays you've had. The interaction between chronological, biological and psychological age was demonstrated by a ground-breaking experiment carried out in 1979 by Professor Ellen Langer of Harvard University.[2]

Professor Langer wanted to research whether changing old people's mindsets could have direct positive physical effects on their wellbeing. She took a group of men in their late seventies and eighties and told them that they would be taking part in a week of reminiscence. They were not told that they would be taking part in an experiment on ageing. She split them into two groups, and whilst one group did indeed spend the week reminiscing about 1959, the other group was put in a carefully constructed time-warp environment for one week. They were surrounded by sights, sounds and sensations that they had experienced when they were younger. They were not helped with any of their day-to-day tasks and were encouraged to manage as they had back in 1959. There were no aids or gadgets designed to help older people. They discussed news of the time in the present tense, watched films and listened to the music of that year.

Professor Langer took physiological tests before and after the experiment and found the improvements to be significant. There was a measurable improvement in their blood pressure, speed of movement, gait, dexterity, arthritis, cognitive abilities and memory. Amazingly, their eyesight and hearing also got better in the one week of the experiment. Both groups showed improvement, but the group that was in the 1959 environment showed the most.

Professor Langer believes that because the men were encouraged to be more independent and no longer thought of themselves as old, their bodies began to respond to their new, younger mindset and started to become physiologically younger.

> *My own view of ageing is that one can, not the rare person but the average person, live a very full life, without infirmity, without loss of memory that is debilitating, without many of the things we fear.*
>
> – Professor Ellen Langer

A repeat of Langer's study was undertaken for the BBC in 2010; a group of ageing celebrities in their seventies and eighties were put into an environment from the 1970s. Using similar protocols, the results mirrored the original experiment, showing measurable improvements in physical and cognitive function, physiological factors that are widely supposed to decline with age.[3]

The A.G.E. Reframe

One of the simplest ways to begin shifting your perception of ageing is to catch yourself *in the moment:* when an unhelpful thought arises, when self-judgement creeps in or when a situation triggers old conditioning. You don't need hours of reflection to begin changing your inner dialogue. Just a few conscious breaths and a gentle reset can make a meaningful difference. That's why we created the A.G.E. Reframe. Our intention was to devise an easy-to-remember way to help you pause, reflect and reframe your thinking in a way that feels grounded, grateful and empowering. You can use it anytime, anywhere as a quick mindset shift. We have included a worksheet in the Companion Guide for when you have the chance to slow down, tune in and turn insight into action. It guides you through the A.G.E. Reframe in a structured, reflective way. It helps you notice limiting thoughts, reconnect with gratitude and consciously choose a more supportive and empowering mindset.

A – Acknowledge

Notice the thought, comment or situation that triggered your reaction. It might be something you said to yourself like "I'm too old for that," a birthday card that jokes about getting older, an advert for stair lifts aimed at older people or a moment of comparison when you hear a comment referring to someone as "still looking amazing for their age." Just pause and name it: What am I telling myself about ageing right now?

G – Gratitude

Shift your focus to appreciation. What has growing older brought you? Experience? Resilience? Wisdom? Perhaps meaningful relationships, life lessons or a deeper sense of self. Even a simple *"I'm grateful to have reached this age"* helps shift your perspective.

E – Empower

Now choose a more supportive perspective. What would an empowered view of ageing sound like? For example:

- "I'm open to seeing ageing differently, even if I'm not there yet."

- "I'm growing into who I truly am."

- "My life experience is a strength."

- "I have more clarity now about what really matters."

Use this step to actively replace fear or doubt with something grounded, hopeful and self-affirming.

Suggestions for Practising the Reframe

- Use it in the moment when a disempowering thought about ageing is triggered.

- Create a new daily habit when looking in the mirror, for example, when you brush your teeth. Looking into a mirror helps you literally face up to your thoughts and consequently connect more deeply with yourself. It turns the words from a thought into something you feel, see and begin to believe.

- Write down a few empowering phrases in a journal or on sticky notes to remind yourself of the new mindset you're choosing. Keep it in your diary, on your desk, in your wallet or somewhere you'll see it every day until it feels an integral part of your outlook.

- If you like, turn it into a mini-ritual, something you come back to whenever you feel the old messages creeping in.

Applying the A.G.E Reframe

Between June 2021 and July 2022, there was only one month when we didn't attend a funeral. With the exception of one person who died suddenly, all the others had suffered horrible symptoms in the last few months of their lives. We sat at bedsides, held hands and witnessed the fear and quiet courage of people coming to terms with the time they had left. It was deeply humbling and emptied our emotional tanks. It's easy to tell ourselves, "That won't happen to me." But as we looked at the patterns in our own family histories – our grandparents, all four of our parents having struggled with illness in later life – we couldn't ignore that we might be facing a similar path.

After learning that a school friend had died, Sue felt a sharp jolt of disbelief. It wasn't just sadness; it was the unsettling realisation that someone she had once sat next to in classes for seven years and shared teenage dreams with was suddenly…gone. The shocking news stirred up so many thoughts and questions. "How was her mum coping?" She must have been so proud when she was made Head Teacher, a perfect role for her confident, resilient and forthright daughter. "How can someone in their fifties, so dedicated to their career and family and always appearing to be fit and healthy, die so suddenly?" "Where did all those years go?" "I should have met up more frequently" and "When will it be me that school friends are telling each other that I'm no longer here?"

Even though the experience of attending so many funerals in a short space of time was perspective-building as it makes you value every day, we didn't realise the cumulative effect of how it was shaping our outlook on ageing. Every funeral was a wake-up call and reminder of what was potentially ahead, a stark reminder of mortality. Forgetting why we had walked into a room sparked, "Is this the start of dementia"? A rotten headache, "Is this a brain tumour?" It wasn't until we had a few months off from attending funerals that we realised how much impact they had had on us. Reminded of the quote in *The Power of Now* by Eckhart Tolle, "Worry pretends to be necessary but serves no useful purpose," we realised we needed to chip away at replacing these fear-based thoughts and find a way to do something simple and easy to integrate into our day. And that's where the A.G.E. Reframe originated from. We started by tuning into our inner dialogue, noticing any thoughts or feelings that weren't helpful, being appreciative and choosing more empowering language.

Applying the A.G.E. Reframe has helped us be more observant of what we're thinking and feeling in that moment and consciously choose a different thought. Over time, this simple practice has changed our perception of ageing significantly.

The Changing Paradigm of Time

> *"There's a lot to be said for giving thanks for getting older, when you know what the alternative is."*
>
> – Nigella Lawson

Every stage of our lives brings challenges or rewards. Social media can place a huge amount of pressure on younger people to conform and to compare themselves with others. When older people are asked what they would tell their younger selves, one of the key themes is around self-acceptance, embracing their uniqueness and not being concerned about what others think. People whose parents died at a young age are often more grateful for having the chance to be old, particularly when celebrating that first birthday that their parents didn't reach. So when Sue hears people say, "I hate getting old," she makes sure they will never repeat that statement to her again!

Feeling grateful for the number of years we have had on the planet is a great basis for valuing our older years. Interviews with surviving military personnel from the Second World War always include how grateful they are to have had the opportunity to live a long life. In an interview with the Radio Times when she was 102, Selma van de Perre, a resistance fighter who undertook dangerous missions and lost her family in concentration camps, said, "When people say they don't want to get old, I say, 'If you're healthy enough, it's very good.'"

Reaching our older years in the 21st century is something to be very grateful for. Later years are more commonly framed as an opportunity for personal growth, fulfilment and wellbeing. Research shows that people often feel happier and more at peace with themselves as they age.

Scientific studies are continually uncovering new evidence that how we age is not based on our date of birth. It's about how we live: the food we eat, the way we move, how we manage stress and how we think. These discoveries are rewriting the rulebook on what's possible in our later years. For example, it's empowering to learn that our genes are not our destiny. We may have inherited certain risks from our parents, like heart disease or diabetes, but scientists now understand that our lifestyle choices can determine how genes are expressed. That means we have much more control over our health than we ever thought.

For a long time, it was believed that we stopped making new brain cells in adulthood. But scientists have now discovered something called neuroplasticity, the brain's ability to adapt, form new connections and even grow new cells well into later life. This means memory, creativity and mental clarity can continue to thrive as we age. Learning a new skill, trying a different routine, practising mindfulness or simply staying curious can all help keep the brain flexible and sharp.

That said, it's not always easy. You might feel resistance to stepping outside of your comfort zone, worry that it's "too late," or fear that your memory isn't what it once was. Starting something new can feel daunting, especially if you haven't challenged yourself in that way for a while. But the good news is, you don't have to make big changes overnight.

Start small. Try brushing your teeth with your non-dominant hand. Take a different route on your regular walk. Learn a new word each week or learn ten words in a new language. Do a puzzle, play a musical instrument or try a new recipe. Even tiny changes can spark new neural pathways.

The key is to stay open and curious. Your brain is far more capable than you may think. The more you use it, the stronger and more adaptable it becomes.

In the Resources section of our website www.getstrongfitandhappy.com, you'll find studies that provide convincing and empowering evidence that declining health as we age is not inevitable.

Studies such as these are helping to create a huge shift in perception, redefining ageing from a linear decline to a spiral of growth, where each stage of life brings unique challenges and profound rewards. Embracing ageing reflects a cultural transformation that celebrates continuity, adaptability and lifelong potential.

Final Thoughts

Many of the beliefs we hold about ageing aren't our own. They've been passed down through stories, stereotypes and social cues so familiar, we often don't question them. But as we've seen, these perceptions are not fixed truths. They're learned ideas, shaped by language, media, culture and the roles we see played out around us.

The good news is that anything learned can be unlearned. Once we become aware of the scripts we've absorbed, we're free to rewrite them. By consciously examining the stories we've been told – and the ones we continue to tell ourselves – we open the door to a more empowering and expansive view of what it means to grow older.

In the next chapter, we'll explore just how important our thoughts, feelings and perceptions are when it comes to ageing.

"We don't see things as they are, we see them as we are."

– Anaïs Nin

CHAPTER 2
Mind-Body Connection

"Because the mind influences every cell in the body, human ageing is fluid and changeable; it can speed up, slow down, stop for a time and even reverse itself."

– Deepak Chopra

Most of us are aware of the mind-body connection in the sense that we'll get "butterflies" in our stomach when nervous or blush when we feel embarrassed. What we often overlook is how integral the mind-body connection is to our vitality and its long-term impact on our health.

We were exceptionally excited about writing this chapter. It's a subject that has fascinated us for decades, and yet we're still learning. We'll share some examples of how we have applied this concept to improve our own health. We'll also share one of many incredible stories of people who have tapped into its power and transformed their health, overcoming life-threatening illnesses to become vibrantly healthy again. We hope this will inspire you to integrate mind-body practices into your vitality toolkit.

To lay the foundations of why it's so important, we'll first take a quick look at the science behind it. If you're anything like us and you understand the rationale for something, you're far more likely to take it on board rather than just see it as another health tip you need to add to your long To Do list.

Whether you're new to the concept of the mind-body connection or are familiar with its power, review the practical tips throughout the chapter and choose the ones that resonate with you. You'll be amazed by the transformations you'll achieve by incrementally integrating a few practices at a time. This builds on what you saw in the last chapter with Ellen Langer's research clearly showing how changing older people's mindset has direct positive physical effects on wellbeing. The more we understand the impact of the mind-body connection, the more we'll be able to live and breathe the benefits, whatever age we are.

But first, some science and history....

From a Biological Machine to the Quantum Body

For much of history, the human body was seen as a mystical or spiritual entity, governed by unseen forces. During the Scientific Revolution, a radical shift occurred. René Descartes, a 17th-century philosopher, argued that the mind and body were distinct entities; a perspective that dominated Western medicine for hundreds of years.

Together with Isaac Newton's groundbreaking work in physics, revealing that the universe operates like a giant machine governed by precise mathematical laws, this mechanistic view was extended to the human body. It was seen as a biological machine made up of separate parts that break down with wear and tear and that could be analysed, fixed or replaced. Disease, in this model, was treated as a mechanical failure rather than an imbalance of energy, environment or consciousness.

Newton's physics led to tremendous advancements in medicine, such as the rise of anatomy and physiology, studying the body like a machine with separate systems. The development of surgery and pharmaceuticals focused on fixing broken parts.

While this approach led to life-saving medical breakthroughs, it also created limitations:

- The body was treated as separate from the mind and emotions.
- Healing focused on symptoms rather than root causes.
- Energy, consciousness and self-healing mechanisms were largely dismissed.

Beyond the Machine:
The Quantum Paradigm

By the 20th century, the discovery of Quantum Physics shattered the classical view of the body as a rigid machine, revealing a far more dynamic and interconnected reality:

- Matter is not solid but composed of vibrating energy fields. At the most fundamental level, we are not fixed physical structures but constantly shifting fields of energy, information and subatomic particles, continuously interacting with our environment.

- The observer affects reality, meaning consciousness plays a role in shaping the physical world. Experiments in quantum physics demonstrate that the mere act of observation influences the behaviour of particles. In the same way, our thoughts, emotions and intentions shape the body's biochemical responses, reinforcing the mind-body connection at the deepest level.

- The body is not just a machine but an intelligent, self-organising system. Rather than operating like a pre-programmed mechanism, the body is deeply influenced by energy, emotions and consciousness, responding dynamically to our internal and external environment.

Quantum physics has enabled us to see the body as more than just a machine and encouraged a more holistic understanding and more dynamic perspective, one where our thoughts, emotions and environment actively shape our health, longevity and overall vitality.

A few years ago a client of Stu's had been told she would need to undergo surgery to remove part of her large intestine and was scared she may need to rely on a colostomy bag. She was feeling powerless until Stu explained the role that our thoughts, emotions and beliefs have in our body's capacity to heal. Combined with some changes in her diet, her symptoms disappeared. Tests carried out on the next hospital visit astonished her consultant, who was able to confirm that she no longer needed surgery.

Levels of Connection:
From Cells to Atoms to Energy

To truly grasp how thoughts, emotions and beliefs influence our physiology, we need to explore the body at different levels:

The Cellular Level: Intelligence Within Each Cell

At the cellular level, your body is constantly regenerating and responding to your inner and outer environment. You create millions of new cells every second, and each cell is influenced by your thoughts, feelings and even your perceptions of the world.

As you'll remember from Chapter 1, genes do not determine our destiny. Groundbreaking research in epigenetics by Dr. Bruce Lipton, author of *The Biology of Belief* showed that cells are not controlled solely by DNA.[1] Instead, they respond to signals from their environment, including the energetic and emotional signals generated by your thoughts, feelings and beliefs. Positive thoughts, gratitude and self-compassion can signal your cells to shift into repair, regeneration and vitality mode.

In contrast, chronic stress and negative beliefs can keep the body in a state of heightened alert, triggering the release of stress hormones like cortisol and adrenaline. Over time, this prolonged stress response can suppress immune function, accelerate ageing and disrupt the body's natural ability to heal and thrive.

By consciously shifting our inner dialogue and cultivating positive emotional states, we can create a biochemical environment that supports cellular renewal, resilience and long-term wellbeing.

The Atomic Level: You Are Mostly Empty Space

If you zoom in even further, beyond your cells, you reach the atomic level. Here, things get even more fascinating. Atoms, which make up all the matter in your body, are more than 99.999999999999% empty space.

The classical view of the atom was similar to the planets rotating around the sun. Electrons were thought to circle round the nucleus in a predictable pattern. Instead, they exist as vibrating energy waves that pop in and out of existence, influenced by observation and intention. This discovery, made by pioneers of quantum physics like Niels Bohr and Werner Heisenberg, shattered the old mechanistic view of the body and revealed that we are fundamentally composed of energy, not solid matter.[2] Therefore, at the atomic level, your body is a dynamic field of energy and information, constantly interacting with the energy around you. This means that your thoughts, emotions and intentions don't just affect your mind; they ripple down to the atomic level, influencing your entire energetic field.

The Quantum Level:
The Power of Intention and Coherence

Quantum physics also reveals that the observer influences reality. This phenomenon is aptly known as the observer effect, in which the simple act of observation affects the behaviour of quantum particles, suggesting that consciousness itself plays a role in shaping physical reality, including your health and wellbeing. Practices like meditation, breathwork and heart coherence (as studied by the HeartMath Institute) help bring your energy field into balance, creating measurable changes in heart rate, brain waves and cellular function.[3] When your thoughts and emotions are aligned in a state of coherence, your body's systems (nervous, immune and endocrine) function more harmoniously. This can enhance vitality, slow the ageing process and support healing at the deepest level.

Mind-Body Practices to Explore

These small, actionable steps can help align thoughts and energy with vitality and wellbeing:

Practise Gratitude to Influence Cellular Repair

- Each morning or before bed, list three things you appreciate about your body, such as "My heart beats for me" or "My lungs breathe effortlessly."
- Say thank you to your body out loud when you notice strength, resilience or healing.

Visualise Your Body as a Vibrant Field of Energy

- Before sleep or upon waking, imagine each cell in your body glowing with health and renewal.
- If an area of your body feels weak or painful, picture it bathed in golden light or vibrant energy, healing from within.

Heart Coherence Breathing

- Place your hand on your heart and breathe in for 5 to 6 seconds, out for 5 to 6 seconds while focusing on feelings of love, gratitude or appreciation.

- Envisage your heartbeat syncing with feelings of calm and inner strength.

Rewire Your Self-Talk for Vitality

- Replace limiting beliefs such as "My joints are stiffening up" with empowering ones like "Every day, I move with greater ease and strength."
- When you catch yourself focusing on aches or fatigue, pause and redirect your attention to something your body is doing well.

Use Movement as a Message to Your Cells

- Even small movements signal renewal – stretch when you're waiting for the kettle to boil, dance, walk barefoot on grass, sweep up the leaves in the garden, walk when chatting on the telephone.
- Try Tai Chi, Qi Gong or yoga, imagining energy flowing freely through your body.

Immerse Yourself in Regenerative Environments

- Surround yourself with images and stories of vibrant ageing.
- Follow people who inspire you with their ageless energy and approach to life.
- Spend time in nature, absorbing its rhythm of renewal and vitality.

Soothe Your Nervous System to Support Healing

- Engage in gentle self-massage, tapping or progressive muscle relaxation.
- Take a few moments each day to sit in silence, letting your body and mind settle.

Celebrate the Magic of Small, Consistent Changes

- Instead of "all or nothing," focus on small, joyful upgrades to your routine.
- Track how each new practice makes you feel over time, rather than looking for immediate changes.

Meditate on Your Interconnectedness

- Reminding yourself that you are not just a physical body, but a dynamic, energetic being.

Integrating These Practices

As straightforward as these practices are, don't feel you're on your own if you come up against resistance or challenges when trying something new like this. It's completely normal, especially when it involves tuning into your body and changing long-held thought patterns.

You may feel a bit strange talking to your body if this is new to you or struggle to believe the new words you're saying. You might feel impatient if changes don't come quickly or doubt whether something so simple can really make a difference. Please know that this is all part of the process.

- **Celebrate progress, not perfection.** If you forget one day, simply return the next. There's no such thing as failure here. Every time you return to your body with love or awareness, you're building a new relationship with ageing, one moment at a time.

- **Notice the subtle shifts and release the pressure to "feel it" immediately.** These practices often work beneath the surface, bringing more calm, more resilience or a softening of the way you speak to yourself. Keep a small journal or note on your phone to track tiny wins or moments of insight.

- **Allow space for your emotions.** Sometimes these practices stir up unexpected feelings: sadness, frustration, grief or even resistance. That's not a sign you're doing it wrong; it's often a sign that something meaningful is shifting. Allow yourself to feel what arises without judgement. You can simply say, "This is part of the process," and breathe through it.

- **Let go of comparison**. You may read stories of people who swear by meditation or breathwork and feel discouraged if your experience isn't the same. Remember, your path is unique. These practices aren't a race or a performance; they're invitations. Show up exactly as you are and trust that's enough.

- **Expect natural ebbs and flows.** Some days you'll feel deeply connected; other days, you may feel flat or distracted. This is the rhythm of life, not a setback.

On low-energy days, consider choosing the gentlest version of a practice: a single breath, a kind word to your body and know that it still counts.

- **Trust the cumulative effect.** Think of these practices like filling a cup with drops of water. One drop might not seem like much, but over time, they add up. The benefits may unfold quietly, showing up as more patience, improved sleep, supportive self-talk or a renewed sense of possibility.

Remember, this isn't about achieving some perfect "ageless" state. It's about building a more loving, trusting and hopeful relationship with your body and your life as you grow older. Every small step counts.

This simple approach is exactly what made a difference in the life of a client of Stu's. He had found it difficult to keep a healthy weight in his forties and fifties, and Stu could clearly sense shame, guilt and despondency during their coaching sessions. This mindset had led to him to approach exercise as a chore that he either put off or went all out and ended up injured.

Stu asked him to tune into his inner dialogue and replace self-critical thoughts with more supportive ones, as if he were helping a valued friend. Stu also suggested keeping a notebook by his bed and writing down three things he appreciates about his body and photos of how he'd like his body to look. During exercise sessions, Stu reminded him to visualise his muscles working and getting stronger.

Over the course of two weeks, these simple practices changed his approach to exercise. Instead of seeing it as a chore, he looked forward to it, which meant that he was more consistent in his practice. In six months, he lost 20 kilograms and significantly changed his body shape, even gaining a flat stomach for the first time in years. This amazing achievement gave him more momentum for his longer term fitness and helped him be aware of what's possible.

Our Thoughts and Emotions Matter

While quantum physics has transformed our understanding at the cellular and atomic levels, neuroscience, a field much closer to everyday experience, has provided profound shifts in mind-body science.

Neuroplasticity

For much of the 20th century, scientists believed that the brain was a fixed and unchanging organ, incapable of generating new neurons after childhood. It was widely accepted that once brain cells were lost, they were gone forever. Research in neuroplasticity has proven that the brain remains adaptable throughout life, capable of rewiring itself in response to thoughts, emotions, experiences and behaviours. Even more astonishing is the discovery of neurogenesis: the brain's ability to create new neurons, particularly in the hippocampus, a region essential for memory and learning.

This means that how we think, what we do and how we care for ourselves directly shapes our brain's structure and function.

Movement, meditation, meaningful learning and deep social connections are not just good for the mind, they actively stimulate the growth of new neural pathways, keeping the brain resilient and vibrant at any age.

Neuroscience has shown us that thoughts and emotions are not abstract forces; they are biochemical signals that shape the body's physiology. Stress, for example, can shrink the hippocampus, while practices like gratitude and mindfulness stimulate neuroplasticity, enhance immune function and promote cellular repair. In this way, our mental state directly influences our physical health, proving that the way we think and feel isn't just in our heads; it's woven into our entire being. Consequently, ageing does not mean inevitable decline. It means endless opportunities for growth, renewal and transformation.

> **Play With New Sensory Inputs to Keep Your Brain Youthful**
>
> - **Daily habits.** Try brushing your teeth with your non-dominant hand to strengthen neural pathways or balance on one leg.
> - **Learn something new.** Doing so activates new brain connections. Try out a new language or musical instrument, take up a new hobby or learn to play a new game.
> - **Change your routine.** Take a different route on your walk, try a new recipe at least once a week or try new cuisine.
> - **Revisit childhood simple pleasures.** Colour, doodle, build something with your hands or play a simple puzzle game. Creativity and play are powerful brain enhancers.

> - **Listen to music mindfully.** Music stimulates multiple areas of the brain at once. Try listening to a new genre or paying close attention to the layers of sound.
> - **Practise "pattern interrupts."** If you always sit in the same spot at dinner, choose a different chair. These small changes tell your brain, "Something new is happening," which enhances alertness and flexibility.

It's completely natural to experience resistance to these kinds of exercises. Our brains are designed for efficiency, so they favour the familiar even if the familiar isn't always helpful. Trying something new requires extra energy and attention, which the brain may initially resist. But it's precisely in these moments of gentle disruption that growth, renewal and new neural connections can begin to form. Here are some common challenges:

"This feels weird; I'm not sure it's working."

New brain pathways take time to form. At first, you might feel clumsy, forgetful or unsure of the point. That's a sign your brain is paying attention, and that growth is happening beneath the surface.

Try this: Turn it into play. Laugh at the awkwardness. Be curious rather than critical. Even a few moments of novelty each day can stimulate brain plasticity and spark up your routine.

"I'm too set in my ways to change now."

It's a common belief and entirely untrue. Although the brain loves efficiency it also wants novelty and stimulation, no matter your age. The key is starting small and choosing something that feels doable.

Try this: Pick one fun, low-pressure change to your day: a new spice in your cooking or a new song to dance to while doing the housework. Let change feel light and nourishing rather than like a chore.

The Reticular Activating System

> *"To despair of growing old makes you grow old faster, while to accept it with grace, keeps many miseries, both physical and mental from your door."*
>
> – Deepak Chopra

The Reticular Activating System (RAS), described in "The Chimp Paradox" and originally discovered in 1949 by neuroscientists Giuseppe Moruzzi and Horace Magoun, is a network of neurons in the brainstem that plays a vital role in attention, wakefulness and perception.[4] It acts as a mental filter, determining which information is prioritised by the brain. This explains why, after deciding to buy a red VW Polo, you suddenly start seeing them everywhere; you've unconsciously signalled to your RAS that red VW Polos are important. It's useful to see the RAS as a searchlight; whatever you focus on, it highlights.

The same principle applies to how we perceive ageing. If we consistently focus on signs of decline, the RAS amplifies that perception and your brain will find more proof of it, reinforcing the belief that ageing equals deterioration. However, by consciously training the RAS to seek vitality and wellbeing, we can shift our brain's focus, prioritising evidence of strength, resilience and renewal. In this way, what we repeatedly notice shapes our reality, not just psychologically, but biologically, reinforcing the mind-body connection.

> **Activities That Use the RAS to Shift Your Mindset**
>
> - Daily practice: Ask yourself empowering questions such as:
>
>   "Where do I feel strong, flexible or energised today?"
>
>   "What signs of health and vitality can I notice in myself?"
>
>   "Who do I know who embodies ageing with energy and enthusiasm?"
>
> - Keep a vitality journal where you record daily moments of feeling strong, capable or connected to life.
>
> - Be mindful of who you socialise with. If you're spending the majority of your time with people who are constantly moaning about getting older and their health issues, it's draining and much harder to disconnect from their vibe!
>
> - Use visual cues. Place images of vibrant people or quotes on ageless living, where you'll see them daily.
>
> - Prime your mind before sleep. Review moments in your day where you felt strong, joyful or connected.
>
> - Create a "Vitality Vision." Imagine yourself thriving at 80, 90 and beyond. How do you move, feel and live? Your brain will begin working toward that vision.

The Chemistry of Emotion: Feelings Shape Your Biology

"Health and happiness are often mentioned in the same breath, and maybe this is why: Physiology and emotions are inseparable."

– Dr. Candace Pert

Emotions serve as the bridge between the mind and body, influencing everything from neural activity to physical health. The very word "e-motion" hints at its essence: energy in motion, a dynamic force that shapes our thoughts, behaviours and physiological responses. Neuroscience has revealed that emotions are not just fleeting feelings but powerful biochemical signals that influence brain function, immune response and even gene expression. When we experience emotion, neural pathways are reinforced, shaping how we perceive and interact with the world. In this way, emotions are not separate from the body but an integral part of our biological reality, acting as the energetic link that weaves together thought, sensation and experience.

Why Affirmations Without Emotion Aren't Enough

Many people have tried affirmations, repeating positive statements like *"I am healthy, strong and vibrant,"* only to feel frustrated when they don't seem to work. The reason? The human mind operates on two levels:

The Conscious Mind

- This is the rational, analytical part of the brain that makes decisions and sets goals.

- When you repeat an affirmation, it happens at this level.
- It's responsible for 5% of cognitive activity with 40 nerve impulses her second.

The Subconscious Mind

- This vast storehouse holds our beliefs, emotions, past experiences and automatic responses. It drives most of our behaviours, often without us realising it.
- If an affirmation conflicts with deeply ingrained subconscious beliefs, such as "ageing means losing my fitness" or "I'm not as flexible as I used to be" then saying the opposite with mere words won't be enough to create real change.
- The subconscious mind speaks in emotions, images and sensations, not just words.
- It's responsible for 95% of cognitive activity with 40 million nerve impulses per second.

Emotion + Embodiment

For an affirmation to work, it needs emotional charge. If you say, *"I feel youthful and energised,"* but deep inside you feel exhausted and resigned, your subconscious will reject the statement. However, when affirmations are paired with strong emotion and physical engagement, they become more effective.

One powerful way to embed affirmations deeply into the subconscious is EFT (Emotional Freedom Techniques), also known as tapping. We highly recommend "Tap with Brad," the details can be found in the Further Resources section.

Releasing Old Cellular Memories to Rewrite Your Mind-Body Story

Our body stores emotions and memories on a cellular level, meaning that past experiences, especially those linked to fear, stress or limiting beliefs, can be imprinted in our nervous system. EFT is a simple yet profound technique that helps to clear out these old emotional imprints.

EFT combines:

- Tapping on specific acupressure points on the face and body
- Repeating targeted affirmations while engaging with the emotional charge

For example, if someone has deeply held fears about ageing, they might tap while saying: "Even though I've believed ageing means decline, I choose to see this as a time of wisdom, vitality and possibility."

This process interrupts old neural pathways, calms the nervous system and allows the subconscious to accept new, empowering beliefs. Studies show that EFT can reduce cortisol (the stress hormone), release trauma and even shift limiting subconscious programs.

Research continues to validate the physiological benefits of EFT in ways that are particularly relevant to ageing. Dr. Peta Stapleton, a clinical and health psychologist at Bond University, has conducted a number of studies showing that a single EFT session can reduce cortisol levels by an average of 43% – far more than traditional talk-based stress interventions.[5] Since chronic stress is a major contributor to accelerated biological ageing, inflammation, memory decline and immune suppression, anything we can do to reduce stress hormones is critical for maintaining vitality in later years.

In a further study involving over 200 participants, EFT was shown to improve key health markers such as blood pressure, resting heart rate and immune function, all of which play a role in maintaining wellbeing as we grow older.[6] These shifts reflect a rebalancing of the nervous system that supports better sleep, emotional regulation and overall wellbeing. Early neuroimaging studies also suggest that EFT may reduce activity in brain areas associated with fear and stress, potentially helping to shift long-standing anxieties about ageing, loss or decline.

By integrating EFT, or even just gently tapping while speaking affirmations, we communicate with the deeper mind where real change happens. And by lowering stress, boosting emotional balance and reinforcing more empowering beliefs, EFT offers a simple yet powerful way to support healthier ageing.

Linking Ancient Wisdom and Modern Neuroscience

In her groundbreaking book *Molecules of Emotion*, neuroscientist Dr. Candace Pert explores the profound link between ancient spiritual wisdom and modern science.[7] She reveals how the body's energy centres, known as chakras in Eastern traditions, align closely with major nerve hubs along the spine. These areas are not just symbolic; they are rich in tiny messenger molecules that help the brain and body communicate. These molecules, which Dr. Pert called the "molecules of emotion," play a key role in regulating important bodily functions like heartbeat, digestion, hormone balance and breathing.

What this demonstrates is that our emotions are not just abstract feelings that are in our minds; they influence bodily functions at a cellular level and so have a direct effect on our physical wellbeing. When we engage in practices that calm or energise these centres, such as meditation, breathwork or mindful movement, we're not only soothing the mind but also supporting the body's natural ability to restore balance and heal. This is especially powerful when it comes to ageing, as it reminds us that we can actively influence how we feel and function at any stage of life.

The Role of Our Nervous Systems in Ageing

One of the most groundbreaking discoveries in neuroscience is polyvagal theory, developed by Dr. Stephen Porges.[8] This theory doesn't just explain the mind-body connection in broad terms. It gives us a practical, science-backed framework for understanding how our nervous system shapes our wellbeing, resilience and even the way we age.

By exploring how our body detects safety or threat and how we can actively shift between these states, we gain the ability to self-regulate, cultivate inner balance and enhance vitality at every stage of life.

Science shows that our nervous system plays a central role in how we experience and adapt to ageing, influencing everything from stress resilience to immune function, digestion and even longevity itself.

Polyvagal theory helps us understand how our body continuously scans the environment for cues of safety or danger, shaping whether we feel at ease or on edge. Our autonomic nervous system is designed to protect us, but when it perceives threats – real or imagined – our body shifts into survival mode, prioritising defence over connection, healing and vitality.

When this state of heightened alertness becomes chronic, it places a persistent strain on the body, increasing inflammation, disrupting sleep, impairing digestion and accelerating cellular ageing. Over time, stress hormones like cortisol and adrenaline can weaken the immune system, reduce cognitive function and contribute to conditions commonly associated with ageing, such as high blood pressure, metabolic imbalances and reduced resilience to illness.

In contrast, when we cultivate a state of safety and connection, the body shifts into repair and regeneration mode, supporting longevity, cognitive clarity and emotional wellbeing. By learning to regulate our nervous system, we can slow the ageing process, improve vitality and enhance our overall quality of life.

**Triggers and Glimmers:
Navigating the Nervous System for a Life of Vitality**

Triggers are cues that activate our stress response, shifting us into fight, flight or freeze mode. These may be obvious, such as a sudden loud noise or a heated argument or more subtle, like an old memory, a particular tone of voice or even a thought pattern we've carried for years. When triggered, our body remains in a heightened state of vigilance, draining energy from essential functions like digestion, repair and emotional balance. Over time, chronic stress accelerates ageing, weakens our resilience and diminishes our overall wellbeing.

But just as we have triggers that pull us into stress, we also have glimmers: small, often fleeting experiences that signal safety and calm to our nervous system. A warm smile, the sound of birdsong, the gentle rhythm of waves or the feeling of sunlight on our skin – these are all glimmers that activate the ventral vagal state, the part of our nervous system responsible for connection, ease and resilience. The key to embracing vitality in our later years is learning to recognise, minimise and regulate triggers while actively seeking and savouring glimmers. This isn't about avoiding life's inevitable challenges but about training ourselves to shift toward states of safety, trust and openness, even in difficult moments.

Rewiring the Mind-Body Connection

Shifting our nervous system toward ease, resilience and vitality is not a one-time effort. It's a practice that's important to weave into daily life. By becoming more observant of our inner signals, we move from reacting to triggers to learning from them and from passively experiencing glimmers to actively seeking them out.

While the idea of shifting the nervous system toward calm and connection is empowering, it can also be surprisingly challenging at first. For many of us, stress responses have become so habitual that we don't even question them and they feel normal. The body may resist slowing down or the mind may question whether feeling safe and relaxed is truly "allowed." Past traumas, ingrained thought patterns or long-standing emotional habits can make it difficult at first.

Start with small daily practices, like noticing the breath or pausing to appreciate something beautiful. Over time, these will retrain the nervous system. There may be days when triggers take over and the thought of tuning into any glimmers feels impossible. This is completely normal. It's about being patient, being consistent and most importantly, being compassionate with yourself. We've certainly found that some of our triggers took a while to take the hint that they were no longer required!

Sue had been in "pink alert" mode for so long, continuously on tenterhooks waiting for the next issue to arise, she'd forgotten how to relax and rest. When she finally said she'd have a "Dressing Gown Day" the following Sunday, the thought felt like such a decadent treat. However, Sunday came and she could not sit still and all she could think about was all the jobs that needed doing. Researching for Stu's first book, *Get Strong, Get Fit, Get Happy*, we had learned a lot about the role of stress in age-related illnesses.[9] So, as well as knowing she was stressed, she was also worried about the long-term impact of being stressed! A life-long habit of just getting on with it meant Sue continued to ignore the signs her body was telling her. Constantly on edge and with a short fuse, she assigned it to the menopause and just kept going.

She was finally shocked into action when she had some blood tests that showed her DHEA levels, which naturally decline with age, were more indicative of someone in their late seventies rather than someone about to turn 60. Re-reading the report, she had hoped it would say something different. But the results were evidence of years of not looking after herself, and now she was paying the price. Had irreparable damage been done? Was it too late to do anything? Feeling sorry for herself wasn't going to change anything, so she studied the connection between DHEA and ageing. Unfortunately, the links with heart disease, cognitive decline, osteoporosis, cancers and immune function just added to her sense of foreboding and hopelessness. Reminding herself to take one small step forward, she decided she'd look for some simple things she could implement.

Firstly, she tuned into her inner and outer dialogue. She noticed how often she used the word "difficult," so she started to use more empowering language. When Sue discussed this with Isabelle Moreau, her genius coach, who asked a very simple question, "What if life were easy?" This stopped Sue in her tracks, eyebrows raised up to her hairline. "Easy!" That was a concept that did not compute. That was for others, not her. All her life, she never felt good enough and thought she needed to have to work harder than anyone else. She unknowingly lived by the adage, "If you haven't worked hard for it, it's not worth having." The DHEA test results, which are an indicator of long-term stress, were convincing evidence that this approach was not healthy.

What difference would it make to her stress levels if she started to perceive life to be easy? What stopped her from feeling she deserved an easy life that flowed effortlessly? She'd been telling others about incorporating more glimmers in their lives. Why had she not taken her own advice?! There were always more important jobs to do. "Once I've sorted that out or met that deadline, I'll put some time aside for this." All this time, she had perceived it as a "nice to have" rather than a priority; it was always going to end up on the "one day" list, which of course never comes.

Focusing on ten daily glimmers – simple pleasures like walking in the woods, pausing to watch a sunset, listening to the birds when she hangs out the washing rather than thinking about the next job that needs doing, listening to the sound of the sea on a CD when working, savouring the moment when chatting over a cup of tea, listening to an audio book when doing the housework, curling up on the sofa with a magazine or a novel – these have all been revelatory. Every night when she gets into bed, Sue jots down at least 10 glimmers.

This shift hasn't been plain sailing. Triggers, by their very nature, are automatic, instantaneous and take some taming! There were days when the familiar feelings and old patterns stubbornly refused to be replaced, or they'd appear uninvited out of nowhere. Putting time aside for chilling out continued to feel like a rare luxury for a long time. Guilt would creep in when curling up with a book. Progress didn't follow a neat curve; it looped, paused and sometimes slid backwards.

Yet, over time, she noticed something quietly transformational. The calm and centred feeling she once glimpsed only occasionally began showing up more consistently. Not every day, but often enough to trust it was possible, until eventually it shifted towards the norm rather than the exception. Although she wishes she'd learned this lesson much earlier in her life, this hard-won shift has made her more determined to help others let go of stress and feel attuned to their inner sense of serenity.

Here's how you can integrate trigger and glimmer awareness into your everyday routine:

Notice Your Triggers With Curiosity, Not Judgement

Throughout the day, when you feel tension, irritation or unease, pause and observe. Instead of pushing the feeling away, ask yourself:

- What just happened?

- What thought, environment or interaction might have triggered this response?

To dig deeper, consider these common types of triggers:

A dishonoured value – Did something go against a deeply held belief or principle?

Examples:

- You value respect, but someone dismissed your opinion.
- You believe in openness and transparency, but you interacted with someone who was deceitful.

A self-limiting belief – Did a thought reinforce an old fear or insecurity?

Examples:

- "I'm not good enough."
- "I should be further ahead by now."

A past experience resurfacing – Did this situation remind you of a past wound?

Examples:

- Feeling dismissed may trigger memories of not being heard as a child.
- Feeling out of control may echo a time when you felt powerless.

Sensory or environmental cues – Did something in your surroundings shift your nervous system?

Examples:

- A certain smell, sound or place triggered an emotional response.
- A cluttered space made you feel overwhelmed.

Interpersonal dynamics – Did someone's tone, body language or energy affect you?

Examples:

- A friend's lack of response made you feel rejected.
- Someone's stress rubbed off on you, shifting your mood.

Unmet needs – Did this moment highlight something you're lacking right now?

Examples:

- You're exhausted and need rest, but you keep pushing through.
- You crave connection, but friends and family feel distant.

Instead of seeing triggers as obstacles, treat them as messengers guiding you toward what needs attention or healing.

Transition Triggers to Reset

Once you recognise a trigger, take a moment to reset your nervous system:

- Take three slow, deep breaths, emphasising a longer exhale.//
- Place a hand on your heart or take a grounding walk.
- Remind yourself: "This is just my nervous system responding to protect me"

Actively Seek and Savour Glimmers

Just as we recognise triggers, we can train ourselves to notice and amplify glimmers – small, positive cues that signal safety and connection. These can be moments of warmth, beauty or resonance that bring ease to your nervous system and uplift your state of being. When you find a glimmer, pause and let it sink in. Hold onto the feeling for a few extra seconds. This strengthens your brain's ability to return to states of ease more often.

a. **Sensory glimmers** – Pleasant sensations that signal comfort and grounding:

- Sight – watching the clouds drift by, branches of trees swaying gently in the breeze, sunrises, the beauty of the sky at dusk, sunsets, candlelight, watching snow fall or the flicker of flames of a winter fire
- Sound – birdsong, breeze in the trees, gentle waves ebbing and flowing on the shore, the trickling sound of a stream, laughter

- Smell – scent of fresh flowers, coffee, newly cut lawn, favourite food being cooked, smells that remind you of home

- Taste – first sip of a velvety and sweet hot chocolate, joy of savouring your favourite meal, salty lips when walking by the sea

- Touch - the warmth of the sun on your skin, the feeling of soft fabrics, a warm bath or walking bare feet on grass, a loving hug, holding a hot mug of tea.

b. **Relational glimmers** – Cues of safety and connection with others:

- A warm smile or a friendly face
- A favourite photo of a loved one
- A heartfelt conversation or laughing with a friend
- Making eye contact with someone who sees and acknowledges you
- Feeling the presence of a pet or receiving affection from an animal
- A driver of a car putting their hand up to thank you for letting them through a gap

c. **Movement and rhythm glimmers** – Activities that soothe the nervous system:

- Swaying, dancing or gentle rocking motions
- The rhythm of deep, slow breathing

- Walking in nature and syncing with its natural pace
- Engaging in repetitive, rhythmic activities like knitting, drumming or humming

d. **Creative and expressive glimmers** – Moments of flow and engagement:

- Writing, painting or playing music
- Singing, chanting or listening to a favourite song
- Watching a sunset or absorbing the colours of nature
- Reading poetry, inspiring quotes or an uplifting book

e. **Spiritual or mindful glimmers** – Inner moments of peace and meaning:

- Feeling awe or gratitude for something bigger than yourself
- Practising meditation or breathwork
- Reciting affirmations that resonate with your heart
- Engaging in acts of kindness or service

End the Day With Reflection

Before bed, take a minute to ask yourself:

- What triggered me today, and what did I learn from it?
- What glimmers did I experience, and how did they shift my state?

This simple practice rewires your brain over time, helping you re-charge your resilience, sharpen your self-awareness and feel attuned to what truly matters in everyday life.

Collate Themes Over Time

On a weekly or monthly basis, take a step back and reflect on patterns:

Keep a Triggers and Glimmers Journal

Keeping a notebook handy to record your triggers and glimmers is an extremely effective way of reviewing them objectively and a motivating way to show your progress. It's like being a new parent. As you're there every day, you may not notice how much your child is growing. But when friends and relatives visit, they'll instantly see the changes. In the same way, by keeping a notebook of your triggers and glimmers, you create a way to look back and see how far you've come. You'll begin to notice patterns: what tends to activate your stress response, what consistently soothes it and where you're becoming more resilient. Over time, reviewing your notes provides convincing proof that your nervous system is learning. And as a result, you'll know that your body is diverting energy away from "fight/flight" survival mode to healing "rest/digest/thrive" healing mode. When we first started keeping a journal, we found it useful for being more consciously aware of our trigger-happy triggers! This awareness helped to pre-empt what previously would have been an automatic pilot stress response. It was reassuring to see how the frequency of even the most persistent and stubborn triggers diminished over time.

What's the balance between triggers and glimmers? When most people start to track their reactions, there's often a lot more triggers than glimmers as our protective nervous system prioritises survival and wants to keep us safe. Over time, though, you'll find that your glimmers start to take precedence and as a consequence, you'll be enjoying life more and living in the moment.

Triggers That Keep Showing Up

Is there a recurring theme, such as an old belief, a boundary being crossed or a persistent stressor? Some triggers you may find refuse to go away! If it's a particular person, for example, you may need to forgive them so you can free yourself from them. Willingness to forgive can be tough, though if you see it as setting yourself free rather than condoning their behaviour, it can be a useful reframe. A great Deepak Chopra quote we have found very useful is "You don't forgive someone for their sake. You forgive them for your sake. Don't forgive because they deserve forgiveness. Forgive because you deserve peace."

Persistent triggers can be like deep-rooted weeds in the garden. Some pull out easily, while others have roots that run deep beneath the surface. If we don't tend to them, they keep growing back, often stronger. It isn't just about cutting them down when they appear. It's about getting to the root, loosening the soil and replacing them with plants that you want to have in your garden. And just like a garden, our nervous systems need regular nurturing, pruning and weeding! Those persistent triggers have taken time to take root throughout life so try to be patient and trust that they will diminish over time.

While patience and trust are essential, there are also practical ways to loosen the grip of deep-rooted triggers. While moment-to-moment practices help bring quick relief, some triggers tend to return again and again. These persistent reactions are often tied to long-standing emotional patterns or early life experiences, like deep-rooted weeds in the garden. These persistent triggers can be seen as useful signposts to let us know what needs our focus. They invite us into deeper self-inquiry and more layered healing.

Begin by noticing how these patterns show up in your body – perhaps as a racing heart, tension in the chest or a sudden sense of withdrawal or defensiveness. These are signals that your nervous system is doing its job: trying to keep you safe. Rather than resisting the response, offer yourself curiosity and compassion. You might ask, "What part of me is this trigger trying to protect?" or "When did I first feel this way?" Bringing curiosity and awareness to the root often softens its grip.

You can also begin to reframe the story. Try pairing your insight with a simple affirmation such as, "I understand where this came from, and I am safe now," or "That was then, and this is now." If helpful, jot down your reflections in a journal – not to judge or fix them, but to witness and understand. These insights can also be brought into practices like EFT tapping, as explored earlier, where you can release old emotional imprints layer by layer. Some roots, of course, run deep. If you encounter a trigger that feels too overwhelming, stuck or confusing to work through on your own, consider seeking the support of a skilled practitioner. Trauma-informed counselling, energy healing such as Reiki or one-to-one EFT sessions can provide the safe space and guidance needed to gently untangle what's buried beneath the surface.

Just like a garden, this inner work takes time, patience and care. Each time you engage with the trigger you're nurturing your nervous system so it's better able to return to balance.

Types of Glimmers That Uplift You Most

Are there specific experiences, places or interactions that consistently bring you joy? Are there other experiences that you would like to be intrinsic glimmers – things that you naturally associate with a sense of ease and wellbeing? How could you integrate these into your life?

> **Integrating More Glimmers Into Your Life**
>
> Glimmers are already present all around you, but the key is to train your awareness to notice them and intentionally create more opportunities for them to occur.
>
> - **Daily update of glimmer journal** – Each day, write down a small moment that brought you peace, connection or joy.
>
> - **Curate your environment** – Surround yourself with sounds, scents and colours that evoke calm and happiness.
>
> - **Incorporate micro-moments** – Even a few seconds of feeling a glimmer can shift your state. Pause, breathe and let it sink in.
>
> - **Use glimmers as anchors** – When feeling overwhelmed, recall a past glimmer and visualise it to shift your nervous system toward safety.

Glimmers remind us that safety, joy and connection are always within reach. The more we recognise them, the more we train our nervous system to seek ease, rather than distress, helping us age with greater resilience, peace and vitality.

Small Shifts That Help You Move from Reaction to Regulation More Quickly

When you feel yourself being triggered – whether by stress, frustration or anxiety – it's easy to become stuck in a reactive state. The key to regulation is recognising the shift and actively guiding your nervous system back to a sense of safety and balance. Here are some practical strategies to help you transition from reaction to regulation more quickly:

Engage Your Breath

Your breath is one of the fastest ways to signal safety to your nervous system. Try:

- **Extending your exhale**. Inhale for 4 counts, exhale for 6-8 counts. A longer exhale activates the vagus nerve and calms the body.

- **Box breathing**. Inhale for 4 counts, hold for 4, exhale for 4, hold for 4. This balances your nervous system.

- **Sighing it out**. Take a deep breath in, then let out a long, audible sigh to release tension.

Ground Yourself in the Present

When stress hijacks your system, grounding techniques can bring you back to the present moment:

- **5-4-3-2-1 Method**. Name 5 things you see, 4 things you feel, 3 things you hear, 2 things you smell and 1 thing you taste to bring awareness back to the body.

- **Touch something textured.** Running your fingers over a textured object (fabric, wood or even a stone) can anchor your focus.

- **Press your feet into the ground.** Feeling the connection between your feet and the floor re-establishes stability and presence.

Shift Your Body to Shift Your State

Your nervous system responds to movement, so changing your posture or engaging in gentle motion can help regulate your system:

- **Change your position.** If you're sitting, stand up and stretch. If you're tense, roll your shoulders back.

- **Shake it out.** Gently shake your arms, legs or entire body for a few seconds to release built-up stress.

- **Use bilateral stimulation.** Alternate tapping your hands on opposite shoulders or thighs

- **Engage in rhythmic movement.** Walking, swaying or even rocking in a chair activates the nervous system's calming response.

Use the Power of Sound and Voice

Your vocal cords are directly connected to the vagus nerve, so using your voice or listening to calming sounds can quickly regulate your state:

- **Humming or singing.** The vibration soothes the nervous system and encourages relaxation.

- **Listening to calming music.** Choose slow, rhythmic music to slow your heart rate.

- **Vocal sighing or chanting.** Making an "Ooo" or "Mmm" sound resonates through the body and signals safety.

Create a Glimmer Anchor

Glimmers are small cues of reassurance and connection that can help pull you out of a stress response. When triggered, try:

- **Visualising a past glimmer.** Recall a recent moment of peace or joy and relive it in your mind.

- **Carrying a glimmer object.** A stone, a small photo or a scented hand lotion can serve as a tangible comfort.

- **Looking for a real-time glimmer.** Find one small, safe or beautiful thing in your current environment.

Reframe the Trigger With Self-Compassion

Instead of judging yourself for being triggered, use it as an opportunity to learn:

- **Ask yourself.** "What is my nervous system trying to tell me?"

- **Use self-talk.** "It makes sense that I feel this way. I am safe, and I can move through this."

- **Place a hand over your heart.** This simple act signals self-soothing and self-compassion.

Set Up a Pre-Emptive Regulation Practice

The best way to recover quickly from stress is to have a daily regulation practice, so your nervous system becomes more resilient over time:

- Start your day with breathwork or meditation to set a baseline of calm.

- Move your body regularly to release stored tension.

- Create a "pause habit." Before reacting in stressful moments, take one deep breath and ask, "What do I need right now?"

Over time, these small shifts add up. Each time you catch yourself in reaction mode and use one of these small shifts, you train your nervous system to recover more quickly. Over time, this creates greater emotional resilience, better health and a more peaceful experience of ageing.

Instead of feeling at the mercy of your triggers, you'll develop a toolbox of ways to guide yourself back to balance, one small shift at a time.

Focus on Your Breathing

When it comes to mastering the art of the mind-body connection, there are lots of techniques you can utilise. If you're thinking, "Where do I start then?", we suggest focusing on your breathing.

One of the most powerful ways to influence the nervous system is through the breath. The reason breathing exercises are so effective in creating a sense of calm lies in the deep connection between breath control and neuropeptide production, which are the chemical messengers that influence mood, stress and emotional regulation. The part of the brain that regulates breathing, the brainstem, is the same area responsible for generating neuropeptides.

When we engage in slow, deep breathing, we activate the parasympathetic nervous system, which calms and relaxes us. This directly impacts neuropeptide release, reducing stress-related chemicals like cortisol. At the same time, it also increases calming and feel-good neuropeptides such as oxytocin, which is associated with connection and love and endorphins, our natural pain relievers and mood boosters.

By consciously slowing the breath, we are not just affecting oxygen levels. We are sending biochemical signals to the brain that shift our emotional and physiological state, reinforcing the mind-body connection. This explains why practices like pranayama, coherent breathing and diaphragmatic breathing have been used for centuries to cultivate balance and resilience.

Despite Stu being a Nutritionist, Personal Trainer and Wellbeing Coach, he noticed a decline in his health when navigating a stressful period of his life: supporting ill parents and, in particular, watching helplessly when his fun-loving and physically fit mum's life and identity were scrambled by the debilitating symptoms and indignity of dementia.

From 2019 to 2023, the assessment machine used by our brilliant Functional Nutritionist revealed that Stu's nervous system was gravely out of balance. No vitamin or mineral supplements, no matter how diligently applied, made a dent.

A healthy person's reading falls between 20,000 and 30,000, but Stu's results stubbornly hovered around 358,000 at our annual check-ups. Each time Stu was tested, he waited for the result, hoping that this would be the time when he would see an improvement. But again and again, the result would be the same as before.

As the tests continued, his sense of frustration grew. What did he have to do to get this reading down? He'd invested years of effort into staying fit and healthy, and these numbers felt like a betrayal of his efforts.

He had tried everything he could think of, and each time he introduced a new health strategy into his routine that he hoped would make the difference, he got the same result. He got to the point where he started to dread taking the test and think of any other reasons why his test results were so bad; perhaps the machine was faulty! Yes, that must be it!

Then, in December 2024, after committing to daily meditation for six months and weaving a Wim Hof breathing technique into his morning routine, Stu's next result showed a staggering 91% decrease.

He was elated with the result. He was hoping that the results would be better but could only have dreamt of such a massive drop. Finally! He had managed to resolve what had seemed to be an intractable and deeply concerning problem. Such a massive improvement underlined the synergistic power of combining some simple yet powerful daily practices.

Examples of the Power of Visualisation and Meditation

When studying to be a Louise Hay Wellbeing Coach in 2005, Sue learned how Louise Hay had overcome ovarian cancer through visualisation and meditation techniques. Many of the attendees were on the course as they had applied the techniques to their own health and wanted to learn how to help others do the same. The experiences people shared were awe-inspiring.

It hadn't occurred to Sue before the course that she had unknowingly used these principles decades earlier. In her early twenties during the 1980s, she received a daunting diagnosis of rheumatoid arthritis (RA), which as you may already know, is when the immune system mistakenly attacks the joints causing inflammation, swelling and pain. The rheumatologist warned her that she might be in a wheelchair by the time she reached thirty.

After grappling with the initial shock, she felt a dazed numbness on the train home. Seeing an older woman cycling as Sue walked back in pain from the station made her feel guilty for being envious of her. For a few days she was crushed by the wave of "Why me?" self-pity, worrying about what her future might look like. It was clear to Sue that this was an important wake-up call for having a sense of perspective that enabled her to not get worked up over things that don't matter or can't be changed. She became determined to snap out of victim mode.

She imagined that at that time her immune cells were a bit paranoid, attacking anything in their path including her joints. She would visualise them becoming more chilled out, eagerly zipping through her bloodstream engulfing viruses, toxins and bacteria and seeing her joints as allies not threats. In time her joints were less painful and she had much better range of motion. Years later, during a medical for a new job, tests showed no trace of RA; a result that left her feeling extremely relieved as well as curious. Given that RA is an auto-immune disease, any practice that reduces the stress response is going to support the immune system and minimise inflammation. So, had letting go of unwanted emotions such as resentment and the calming visualisation helped? Even though Sue will never know exactly what enabled her to overcome RA, the experience did make her so much more grateful to her body and, in general, in awe of the human body's amazing capacity to heal.

In another example, we attended an amazing Dr. Joe Dispenza Meditation Course in Barcelona in 2024, where we learnt about many scientific studies that demonstrated the transformative power of meditation in overcoming the most challenging of health issues. One attendee in his seventies agreed to speak on the stage to explain how he was converted from being highly sceptical to being a convert to the importance of daily meditation. Two years previously, he had a 15-cm tumour on his kidney and was seriously ill in hospital. With nothing else to do, he reluctantly read the book on meditation that his son-in-law had left him. Even on days when he was feeling very disheartened and scared about his potentially imminent death, he diligently practised meditation. Six months later, there was no sign of the tumour.

Final Thoughts

The mind-body connection has fascinated us for decades, and we're continually exploring personal development courses to deepen our understanding.

MIND-BODY CONNECTION

A moment that profoundly shifted our perception of the world was in June 1996. Sue had just replaced her old Ford Fiesta, which had no radio, with a VW GT Polo, which had a CD player. This was pure luxury! On our journey down to Dorset, we listened to Deepak Chopra's Magical Mind, Magical Body: Mastering the Mind/Body Connection for Perfect Health and Total wellbeing.[10] One sentence, in particular, opened our eyes to a paradigm shifting new way of thinking: "A photon is to light as an electron is to electricity as a thought is to the mind-body connection."

This reveals that just as photons and electrons are the fundamental forces behind light and electricity, our thoughts shape the intricate interrelationship between mind and body. It serves as a reminder of the immense influence our mindset has on our wellbeing.

We hope this idea inspires you to honour the role your thoughts play in shaping your wellbeing. Next, we'll explore how the wisdom you've gathered over a lifetime – sometimes knowingly, sometimes without even realising it – can become a compass for a more purposeful, fulfilling life.

CHAPTER 3
Life Wisdom

"Just when you think you know something, you have to look at it in another way."

– Dead Poets Society

Many of us expect that wisdom will simply arrive with the passing of the years – yet it doesn't always feel that way. Whether you're still searching for that sense of inner knowing, or you already feel connected with your Wise Elder within, this chapter is here to help you acknowledge, tap into and intentionally apply the life wisdom you've accumulated. By doing so, you can live with greater focus, fulfilment and authenticity in the years ahead.

Imagine stepping into a large library with shelves full of numerous books capturing the wisdom you have acquired throughout your life: strategies learned from experience, insights from challenges and truths that have quietly shaped who you are. Some books are well-thumbed; their lessons etched into your memory and reflective of your day-to-day approach to life. Some may be familiar and in easy reach, but their contents are taken for granted. Others are gathering dust on forgotten shelves, their pages waiting to be re-explored. This chapter invites you to revisit your life's library and bring its wisdom into the present so you can navigate the years ahead with clarity, purpose and fulfilment.

In Japan, "tsundoku" encapsulates the concept of a library of unread books, a poignant reminder of the knowledge and insights we possess yet are not utilising. Thanks to our busyness, we rarely get time to reflect on the profound wealth of wisdom we already possess and focus on how we can consciously apply it to create a life that feels genuinely aligned with who we are. By rediscovering those books, you can transform untapped potential into powerful guidance.

In the next week or so, explore these "life wisdom books" to appreciate the richness of your life. It may be useful to dedicate a journal to capture your reflections using the questions below:

Well-Thumbed Books

These are the lessons etched into your memory and already reflected in daily life.

> What life lessons have become central to how you approach your day-to-day decisions?
>
> Which experiences or memories shaped these lessons?
>
> How do these well-thumbed lessons support or limit you daily?
>
> Are there new perspectives or actions you could explore to deepen your understanding of these lessons?

Familiar Books

These are the lessons within reach but are often taken for granted.

> What knowledge or insights do you often rely on but perhaps undervalue?
>
> How have these familiar lessons shaped your relationships, choices or outlook on life?
>
> Are there ways to rediscover the value of these lessons and apply them more consciously?
>
> What strengths or qualities might you be overlooking because they feel second nature?

Books Gathering Dust

These are the books hidden in faraway shelves waiting to be explored once more.

> Are there past experiences or insights you've set aside that could offer valuable guidance?
>
> What challenges, joys or reflections from your past might you revisit to gain a fresh perspective?
>
> How can you intentionally bring these lessons back into focus and integrate them into your life now?
>
> What untapped wisdom might be waiting for you in areas you've previously overlooked or dismissed?

To build on insights from the wisdom we have acquired in our own lives, it's useful to review the qualities of people we perceive to be wise elders.

Wise Elders and Modern Research

Who comes to mind when you think of a wise elder? Which fictional or real-life figures have guided or inspired you with their life wisdom? Who has taught you profound life lessons, directly or indirectly?

Perhaps it's the Dalai Lama for his spiritual wisdom, compassion and resilience. It may be Nelson Mandela for his ability to forgive and focus on reconciliation. Mother Teresa may be at the top of your list for her profound understanding of human dignity and the power of small acts of kindness.

There may be fictional characters such as Agatha Christie's Miss Marple who embodies humility, patience, objective observation of people without judgement and confidence in trusting her intuition.

Merlin, the wizard of Arthurian legend, is the archetypal wise elder, embodying profound knowledge, foresight, the transformative power of mentorship, adapting to life's inevitable uncertainties and honouring your own moral compass.

Reflecting on the attributes of these wise elders, including compassion, humility, resilience, empathy and adaptability, which ones do you recognise in yourself?

The timeless qualities of wise elders like Mother Teresa, the Dalai Lama, Nelson Mandela, Miss Marple and Merlin are mirrored in modern research on what contributes to a meaningful and fulfilling life. The Harvard Study of Adult Development, initiated in 1938, tracked the lives of over 700 individuals for more than 80 years. It highlighted that strong relationships, built on empathy and understanding, are essential to health and happiness. In line with the Dalai Lama's teachings on interconnectedness, the research showed that this contributed more to greater life satisfaction than wealth or fame.[1]

The Legacy Project conducted by sociologist Karl Pillemer included extensive interviews with over 1,000 older Americans to collate their advice on living well. The findings are detailed in Pillemer's book, *30 Lessons for Living: Tried and True Advice from the Wisest Americans*.[2]

Key lessons included pursuing meaningful work, prioritising relationships and adapting to life's challenges. This theme of adaptability and resilience highlights hallmarks of Mandela's life, as someone who turned personal struggle into a legacy of reconciliation.

Research published in the journal *Psychology and Aging* examined how regret affects quality of life among different age groups. The study found that older adults often experience less regret intensity than younger individuals, possibly owing to a reduced perception of opportunities to change past decisions. However, when older adults do experience intense regret, it can significantly diminish their quality of life. The study suggests that the ability to disengage from unattainable goals and focus on new ones can help manage regrets in later life.[3]

Regrets are, of course, part of being human. From our perspective, if you don't have any regrets, then how fully have you actually lived? Regrets can be powerful life lessons and give us far more direction than those aspects of our lives that we're prouder of or comfortable with. Regrets give us the opportunity to learn a great deal about ourselves, where we've strayed from our values or missed an opportunity to live more fully. We think it's important we review them with curiosity, not judgement. Beating ourselves up about something we can't change saps energy and sucks the joy out of life. At the same time, the heavy emotive charge of regret can lead us to leave them unchecked as they're too painful to think about. They then become an anchor to the past. The guilt or sense of shame that can accompany them can lead us to believe we do not deserve the happiness and possibilities available in the present.

Many conventional and pragmatic views see regret as something we just have to live with as we age, especially if we feel we've "run out of time" to make changes. But we think this is a bit of an excuse! This approach justifies not taking action and keeps us safely in our comfort zone to avoid the risk of making more mistakes. A more empowering view is to see regrets as invaluable, a compass pointing us toward deeper self-awareness and more intentional living from this moment forward. That shift in mindset can be deeply healing.

This is beautifully exemplified by the Dalai Lama, who succinctly encapsulates the power of living with purpose and compassion as a way to transcend regret: "We must each lead a way of life with self-awareness and compassion, to do as much as we can. Then, whatever happens, we will have no regrets."

When we bring self-awareness to our choices and align our lives with what truly matters, regret loses its grip – and the path ahead opens with renewed clarity and hope.

A study by Concordia University explored how perceived control over life regrets impacts wellbeing in older adults. Findings indicate that older individuals who feel they have little control over their regrets tend to experience lower life satisfaction and higher levels of depression. Conversely, those who accept their regrets and perceive some control over their responses exhibit better psychological health.[4]

In her 2011 book *The Top Five Regrets of the Dying: A Life Transformed by the Dearly Departing*, Bronnie Ware, a palliative care nurse, identified five common regrets among the people she supported at the end of their lives:[5]

> "I wish I'd had the courage to live a life true to myself, not the life others expected of me."
>
> "I wish I hadn't worked so hard."
>
> "I wish I'd had the courage to express my feelings."
>
> "I wish I had stayed in touch with my friends."
>
> "I wish that I had let myself be happier."

Although it's sad to think that these are common themes, they provide invaluable insights for us to benefit from so that we can live authentically and meaningfully.

The RESPECT Wisdom Framework

We may not see ourselves as wise elders, yet all of us have assimilated huge amounts of wisdom throughout our lives. When we think about the decisions our younger selves made or the perspectives we had, it's easier to acknowledge how much wiser we are now! It's important that we don't take this for granted but instead acknowledge it and have a keen interest in continually building on it so we can live our lives to the full. The following RESPECT framework was devised to help you explore your life wisdom, recognise its value and highlight areas you may wish to focus on. You may want to use these reflective questions as the basis of a journal. The process of working through these questions will allow you to reaffirm the vast wisdom you've already acquired and help you gain laser-focused clarity on the areas you'd like to improve upon.

R - Relational Wisdom

Insights about relationships and connecting with others. Questions to explore:

> Who are the most important people in my life, and how do I nurture those relationships?
>
> How do I show empathy and understanding in my interactions with others?
>
> Are there relationships I need to mend, strengthen or let go of to maintain my wellbeing?
>
> How do my relationships reflect the values I hold dear?

E - Experiential Wisdom

Lessons learned from life's defining moments and challenges. Questions to explore:

> What life experiences have taught me the most valuable lessons?

How have my successes and failures shaped the person I am today?

Are there areas of my life where I could draw more consciously on past experiences to guide my decisions?

What defining moments in my life hold untapped wisdom?

S - Spiritual Wisdom

Understanding life's deeper meaning and our connection to the universe. Questions to explore:

What gives my life meaning, and how do I connect with it regularly?

How do I find peace and purpose, even in challenging times?

Are there practices or beliefs I can explore further to deepen my sense of spiritual fulfilment?

What roles do gratitude, love or faith play in my daily life?

P - Practical or Intellectual Wisdom

Knowledge and skills gained through education, reading and learning. Questions to explore:

What knowledge or skills have I gained that I use to navigate life's challenges?

> Are there areas where I could seek to learn more to enhance my understanding or problem-solving abilities?
>
> How do I apply what I've learned in meaningful ways to improve my life or support others?
>
> What books, mentors or experiences have significantly shaped my intellectual growth?

E - Emotional or Intuitive Wisdom

Inner knowing and gut feelings that guide decisions and actions. Questions to explore:

> How well do I trust and listen to my instincts when making decisions?
>
> When have I managed my emotions effectively, and what strategies helped me do so?
>
> Are there situations where I need to cultivate more emotional awareness or resilience?
>
> What role does self-compassion play in my emotional health?

C – Challenge, Change, Transformational Wisdom

Growth and insights gained through significant transitions or hardship. Questions to explore:

> What major life changes or challenges have shaped me, and how did I grow from them?

> How do I approach uncertainty and adapt to change in my life?
>
> Are there past challenges I can reflect on to help me navigate current or future transitions?
>
> What have I learned about myself through times of transformation or loss?

T - Timeless or Legacy Wisdom

Lessons and values we wish to leave as our legacy for future generations. Questions to explore:

> What values and lessons do I want to pass on to others, and how am I living those values now?
>
> How do I want to be remembered, and what am I doing today to align with that vision?
>
> Are there ways I can create a positive, lasting impact in my community, family or the world?
>
> What traditions or beliefs do I hope future generations will carry forward?

The Six Human Needs

We first encountered the Six Human Needs in March 2024 during a training course with Robin Banks. It was one of those simple yet profound concepts you occasionally come across that transform the way you see yourself and others. The model was developed by Tony Robbins to expand on Abraham Maslow's hierarchy of needs. Rather than viewing human needs as a sequence,

Robbins proposed that they operate simultaneously, shaping our thoughts, behaviours and emotions. His intention was to help people understand not just what they do, but why they do it.[6] This model provides a practical lens through which to explore how our deepest emotional needs influence the way we live, love and make decisions.

In the RESPECT model, this concept is an example of Practical or Intellectual Wisdom, one that you feel you already know but are not consciously aware of. It helped us enormously to have laser-focused clarity on evaluating the motivation behind what we do and understanding the behaviour of others, which has enabled us to live a more compassionate and fulfilling life.

Understanding the six human needs can transform the way we view life and relationships. It encourages a shift from chasing temporary satisfaction to pursuing deeper fulfilment through balancing what's most important in life. Here's a breakdown of the six needs:

Certainty

We all crave stability and predictability to feel secure. This could mean having a steady job, reliable relationships or even daily routines. However, over-reliance on certainty can limit growth and make life feel mundane. Acknowledging that certainty is often an illusion allows us to embrace change more effectively.

Uncertainty or Variety

Paradoxically, while we seek certainty, we also need variety to keep life exciting and engaging. This could mean exploring new hobbies, meeting new people or trying new experiences. Striking a balance between certainty and variety helps us feel both grounded and adventurous.

Significance

The need to feel important, unique or valued drives many of our actions. It can motivate achievements and self-expression. However, chasing significance at the expense of connection with others can lead to loneliness. Fulfilment comes from balancing this need with love and connection.

Love and Connection

Humans are inherently social beings, seeking love and meaningful relationships. While love and genuine connection bring deeper fulfilment, people often settle for surface-level interactions due to fear, past hurts or sometimes even cultural expectations. Settling for fleeting or shallow connections can lead to feelings of loneliness, disconnection and a nagging sense of emptiness – the opposite of the rich, life-affirming fulfilment that comes from authentic bonds. Learning to prioritise genuine relationships, built on trust, openness and vulnerability, fosters true happiness and enriches life at any age.

Growth

Continuous self-improvement and learning are essential for fulfilment. Like everything in nature, humans thrive when we grow. Growth helps individuals adapt to challenges and feel a sense of progress, making life more meaningful.

Contribution

The ultimate source of fulfilment comes from contributing to something greater than oneself. Acts of giving, whether to loved ones, communities or the world, provide profound joy and purpose. Contribution reminds us that we are part of a larger ecosystem, enriching both ourselves and others.

Being aware of these innate human needs allows us to bring more harmony into our lives. We've found that when we're feeling out of kilter, it's often because at least one of the needs is not being honoured. Taking the time to notice if there's a need that's being neglected, perhaps at the expense of another, it's easier to see what we need to focus on to get back into balance.

In April 2023, we weren't sure if Sue's mum was going to recover after being rushed to the hospital. First of all, we didn't know if she would live through the night. Thankfully, she did – but it was touch and go for a few months. As anyone knows, when you're in this "pink alert" mode, your heart misses a beat every time the phone rings. It's hard to feel settled. We didn't know about the Six Human Needs then, so it took us a while to get our feathers smooth again.

When we experienced a similar period of uncertainty recently, we knew we needed to focus on balancing the unknown with some familiarity. Taking the time to meet up with Sue's family outside of hospital visits helped create a sense of normality. As was the case previously, when time is tight, it's easy to allow getting together to be put on the back burner. But just meeting up for a cup of tea and a chat about nothing in particular helped everyone to feel that reassurance of the familiar, whilst also feeling connected. This is a simple example, but hopefully it demonstrates how the awareness of the Six Human Needs can help you make more intentional choices so you can realign and feel more centred.

From a wider perspective, what made this concept so life-changing for us was also realising how much all the unknowns, constant fears and unexpected challenges we'd faced supporting ill parents had led us to place far too much emphasis on searching for stability and certainty, which in turn had constrained our aspirations and goals. We therefore focused on how to attain a balance between honouring the need for familiarity and embracing the unknown. This impactful quote from Tony Robbins has proved helpful: "The quality of our life is in direct proportion to the amount of uncertainty we can comfortably live with."

We knew that we needed to expand our comfort zone and trust that we'll navigate the inevitable unknowns. In doing so, we were able to unlock our passion for wanting to help people over 50 live their lives to the full. This has given us a huge sense of fulfilment from honouring the 5th and 6th human needs of Growth and Contribution.

Living Life With GRACE

Reflecting on the common regrets of those nearing the end of life – wishing they had lived true to themselves, prioritised relationships, expressed their feelings, worked less and embraced happiness – is a powerful reminder of how to align our lives with what truly matters. These regrets echo the insights from modern research on life wisdom: nurturing meaningful connections, pursuing purposeful activities and cultivating resilience are essential for wellbeing and fulfilment. When viewed through the lens of the Six Human Needs – Certainty, Variety, Significance, Love and Connection, Growth and Contribution – it's clearer to see how these regrets stem from unmet needs or misaligned priorities. We devised the Living with GRACE (Gratitude, Release, Align, Connection and Embrace) model to help people navigate life with clarity, prioritise what matters most and ultimately, live in a way that leaves minimal room for regret.

G - Gratitude

Human need: *Certainty*

Gratitude helps meet the need for certainty by creating a sense of stability and trust in life. When we focus on what we appreciate, we remind ourselves that life provides – even in uncertain times.

R - Release

Human need: *Love and connection*

Releasing resentment and forgiving allows deeper love and connection to flourish. When we let go of the emotional baggage tied to past hurts, we create space for more fulfilling relationships.

A - Align

Human need: *Significance*

Aligning with what matters most ensures that we live authentically and purposefully. When our actions reflect our values, we naturally feel a sense of importance and worth.

C - Connection

Human need: *Love, connection and growth*

Connection meets the need for love and growth. By deepening relationships and building meaningful bonds, we nurture emotional fulfilment and evolve as individuals.

E - Embrace

Human need: *Uncertainty, variety and contribution*

Embracing life's finite nature encourages us to find joy in the unknown and contribute to something greater than ourselves. Awareness of life's impermanence can inspire courage, creativity and giving back.

One of the most profound times Sue applied the GRACE model was on a train journey she'll never forget. Her mum had been rushed to the hospital by ambulance, and the doctors didn't expect her to survive the day. Sue stared blankly out of the window, constantly checking her phone for updates from her sister, powerlessly suspended between two worlds: one with her mum still with us and the unimaginable one that she dreaded living in. Couldn't the train go any faster than this? How many more stations would the train stop at?

The normality of sitting in a train carriage felt surreal. Fellow passengers sipped coffee, scrolled through their phones and flicked through magazines. Trying to make sense of the world and tame her thoughts that were all over the place, she rummaged through her bag and found a notebook and pencil and started writing in the hope of decluttering her mind and to feel something different to this intense numbness yet emotional overload. Then she remembered the GRACE model, which turned out to be a great way to focus her attention and make the journey seem shorter.

Gratitude was easy as Sue had been incredibly fortunate to have such a loving mum and fabulous friend with so many shared moments to be grateful for. What was more challenging was being able to see what she was writing through the tears!

Release was perhaps the hardest. Sue found it hard to let go of the resentment that she felt about this last chapter of her mum's life. They were not the fun-packed and joy-filled final years she had hoped her mum would have. Dementia, heart disease and sepsis had stolen her mum's retirement. What benefit did this resentment bring? How was this going to support her mood when she finally got to be at her mum's bedside? Realising that the resentment wasn't helpful and reframing it as a price for caring made it easier for Sue to release it.

Aligning proved useful for focusing on what would truly matter once she arrived at the hospital: being there for her mum, showing her how much she's loved, supporting her family, etc. Reviewing the long list, it was easy to see the themes of the inner values, such as love, compassion, serenity, empathy, kindness and respect. Reviewing these values gave a sense of clarity and peace.

Connection came naturally. As the train got closer to Margate, Sue couldn't wait to hug her brother and sister, hold her mum's hand and choose her words carefully so she could truly connect with her, bearing in mind this could be the last words she might hear. Thinking about the hospital staff in the Accident & Emergency ward and how dedicated they are to their work, also the people on the train that would probably also at some stage be making a similar journey to see a loved one, helped Sue to connect more widely.

Embrace. Finally, Sue chose to embrace life's fragility. That call earlier from her sister reminded her how unpredictable life is, how every goodbye could be the last and how vital it is to savour every moment. Embracing life's finite nature could not have been more evident that day and helped Sue to think about what she could do to make what could be the final moments of her mum's life as precious as possible.

By the time the train stopped at the station, beyond helping the journey go much quicker, the GRACE model had brought new perspectives to one of the toughest mornings of Sue's life. And now, exactly two years on as we write this, the insights she gained from that train journey remain with her.

Final Thoughts

Life wisdom is the culmination of the lessons, insights and experience we gather over the years. It's the clarity that comes when we step back and see the bigger picture of our lives – the finite nature of time, the importance of relationships and the freedom that comes from letting go of past burdens so we can place our focus on what's most important to us. It's not about having all the answers and never making mistakes. It's not only found in extraordinary events, but also in everyday moments if we take the time to notice. When we pause to reflect on what life has taught us and how we've grown through it, we access a deeper sense of purpose and peace. One valuable lesson that we've learned is not to overcomplicate life or to expect wisdom to be complex or intellectual. As Ralph Waldo Emerson famously said, "The invariable mark of wisdom is to see the miraculous in the common."

If you're anything like us and have a tendency to concentrate on what you haven't yet learnt or mastered, you're clearly not alone. That's why we created the RESPECT framework: Relational, Experiential, Spiritual, Practical, Emotional, Challenge and Timeless. It's designed to help you acknowledge the value of the life wisdom you have already accumulated, and in the process, provide insights for areas you want to work on next.

As you saw, the Six Human Needs framework provides clear signposts to keep us on track for honouring the full spectrum of what it means to be human. We hope the GRACE model – Gratitude, Release, Align, Connection, Embrace – will help you attain a focused balance for living intentionally with purpose, love and a sense of grace.

In the next chapter, we'll explore how we can draw on our life wisdom to guide us through the inevitable challenges of later life, and how those very challenges often deepen and refine that wisdom. We'll also look at practical ways to navigate particularly demanding times whilst staying connected to what matters most.

> *"Wisdom is not a product of schooling but of the lifelong attempt to acquire it."*
>
> – Albert Einstein

CHAPTER 4
Know Thyself

"Ageing is an extraordinary process where you become the person you always should have been."

– David Bowie

Who are you beneath the roles, labels and expectations that have shaped your life? If you haven't had the chance to stop and think about this before, this chapter invites you to rediscover your authentic self and live in alignment with your unique essence. It's a chance to ask: Am I truly being me? Or have I been living someone else's idea of who I should be? You might perceive this to be self-indulgent, or you may be asking, "Isn't it a bit too late to be thinking about this?" or "How do I even know what's right for me anymore?"

As we saw in the previous chapter, the top regret of people at the end of their lives is not having had the courage to live true to oneself, rather than conforming to others' expectations. This is why we believe the lessons in this book are worth focusing on, so you can live the rest of your life on your terms.

We'll explore practical tools and timeless wisdom to help you navigate those "Who am I?" questions with clarity and self-compassion – from understanding your unique mind-body type, to shedding outdated labels, to tuning into your body's own intelligence. We believe knowing yourself isn't a luxury; it's the foundation of true wellbeing, vitality and fulfilment in your later years.

Living Life True to Ourselves

> *"Your time is limited, so don't waste it living someone else's life. Don't be trapped by dogma, which is living with the results of other people's thinking."*
>
> – Steve Jobs

One of the liberating aspects of getting older is feeling less constrained by external expectations – a unique sense of freedom we get as the years go by. We are more aware that we won't be here forever, so we are more inclined to look at what is important to us and, as David Bowie said, become the person you always should have been.

To us, knowing thyself means embracing who you truly are – foibles, quirks, strengths and all – with compassion and honesty. It's about loving yourself unconditionally and making peace with your past, your imperfections and the things that make you uniquely you.

It's also about living in alignment with your values, making choices that honour your physical, mental and emotional needs, and trusting your own inner compass rather than constantly seeking approval or direction from others.

When you know yourself, you stop trying to fit into someone else's idea of how you should age. You start making conscious, informed decisions based on what works for you. You begin to prioritise what nourishes you, what energises you and what lights you up.

In a world full of noise, pressure and one-size-fits-all solutions, knowing yourself is an act of self-respect. It's the foundation for a life of authenticity, vitality and quiet confidence in your later years.

Who Am I?

Throughout life, we accumulate a number of roles which all contribute to how we live our lives. These include:

How we connect with others: son, daughter, partner, parent, grandparent, aunt, uncle, brother, sister, friend, colleague, caregiver.

Working lives: mechanic, plumber, teacher, lawyer, entrepreneur, volunteer.

Hobbies and Interests: Dancer, gardener, runner, potter, painter, cook.

While these roles bring meaning and purpose, they can also create a sense of identity that feels bound to external expectations.

There are also labels that we can allow to define our identity, such as smoker, diabetic, old, etc. The labels we use determine our actions and behaviour. We therefore need to choose these labels wisely.

Shedding any labels that limit us can help redefine ourselves in ways that empower, inspire and reflect the essence of who we truly are. What roles and labels have you collated?

- Which roles give you a true sense of fulfilment?
- Which roles do you play the most?
- Which roles do you play the least?
- Are there any labels that are not serving you well?

A more in-depth exercise to explore this further can be found in the Companion Guide. It's about letting go of old stories and stepping into the person we were always meant to be.

Reputations and Typecasting

The reputation we gain at work can often lead to typecasting, resulting in other strengths and preferences staying backstage. A project manager whom Sue coached had gained a reputation for driving results. His action orientation and strong sense of urgency meant that he was often assigned projects that had lost momentum. He enjoyed the challenge of collaborating with people and working around the obstacles to ensure timely project completion. However, he was not fulfilled in his role.

It was a real "aha" moment for him when he was reminded of his natural propensity for innovation after completing a psychometric profile. His reputation for completing projects meant that he had limited opportunity to honour his innate creativity and enterprising spirit. He spoke to his manager about taking on new projects that address future business needs, giving him a blank canvas and a chance to experiment and generate ideas. This focus on innovation and leading change helped him to be far more fulfilled in his work.

Sue's work with psychometric personality profiles provides numerous examples of the constraints of typecasting and the liberation that comes from people rediscovering their North Star, enabling them to live their lives to the fullest by being true to themselves.

It's worth checking in on the extent to which our innate preferences and motivations are being honoured in our lives.

For many of us over 50, this stage of life presents a powerful opportunity to pause, reflect and realign with what really matters. Without that pause, we risk staying on autopilot – continuing down familiar paths even when they no longer feel right. Over time, this can lead to a quiet sense of disconnection, frustration or the nagging feeling that something important is missing.

Yet when we honour our intrinsic motivators and natural preferences, and draw on our innate strengths and qualities, we automatically feel more centred and fulfilled. Life feels more aligned, and with that alignment comes a renewed sense of meaning, clarity and feeling centred. This is the gift of this stage of life: not just the wisdom to know ourselves better, but giving ourselves more freedom to live in a way that reflects who we truly are.

Taking time to step back and review this regularly is a powerful way to realign with your true self. It helps reveal where your strengths are being fully expressed, and where they might be overlooked. Here are a few questions to guide your reflection:

> Are you relying too heavily on certain skills while underusing other natural talents or attributes?
>
> Which of your strengths do you use and enjoy most regularly?
>
> Which valuable strengths or attributes do you rarely get the chance to draw on?
>
> What qualities or aspects of yourself feel most recognised and valued in your daily life?
>
> Which parts of you feel underused, unseen or in need of more expression?

Connecting With Our True Self

"You may look in the mirror and see a different face, an older face, but the person looking out of those eyes feels ageless. That awareness, that presence you feel, is who you truly are."

– Deepak Chopra

In the film Titanic, the older Rose looks at the mirror that was salvaged from the ship and says, "It looks the same way it did the last time I saw it...The reflection has changed a bit." Despite changes in our physical appearance, there is an unchanging essence that remains constant throughout life.

Although we catch fleeting sight of this true essence when we look in a mirror, we can take it for granted and even lose touch with it as we go through life.

The many roles we play can take precedence over that true sense of self. Exploring who we are beyond labels like "I am a parent" or "I am a diabetic" enables us to rediscover the inner core that has always existed. This core self is not defined by any role, accomplishment or limitation. The more we can connect with this essence and live our lives honouring it, the more fulfilled we will be.

So many people Sue has coached in the later stages of their careers wish they had explored different options earlier. A partner in a law firm felt pressure as a student from his father to follow a career in the legal profession. Though successful in what he had accomplished, he did not feel fulfilled. He was constantly swimming against the tide, not being true to himself, and so was exceptionally stressed. Together with the external pressures of the legal profession, he became ill in his fifties, leading to burnout. Taking the time to explore what motivated him, his core values and innate qualities enabled him to identify a new career that truly fulfilled him. In doing so, his health was restored.

Research shows that the more aligned our lives are with our innate motivations, values and true sense of self, the healthier we'll be.

For example, a 2024 study in Health Psychology Research found that people who prioritised personal values, such as self-care and growth, reported better physical health and lower stress levels, with 60% of participants citing intrinsic motivations as their top driver for healthy behaviours.[1] Similarly, research from Stanford University's Center for Compassion and Altruism Research suggests that living authentically and in alignment with one's core values is associated with lower levels of stress, better immune function and greater life satisfaction.[2]

These findings echo what many wisdom traditions have taught for centuries: when we live in harmony with our true nature, we thrive. Not only mentally and emotionally, but physically too. Dr. Edward Bach encapsulates this beautifully when he says, "Health depends on being in harmony with our souls."

The price we pay in this age of information is that we can be inundated with a ton of data to trawl through, so much so that it can feel overwhelming. This is not helped by the often conflicting information – what was last week's superfood is now to be avoided at all costs. Spinach is full of healthy nutrients, yes, but for people who do not process oxalates efficiently, it can cause lots of unpleasant symptoms and put pressure on the kidneys. The latest trends in health and vitality tend to imply a one-size-fits-all approach, which is rarely the case.

Bio Individuality:
Be True to What's Right for You

"*Some folks have fat feet.*" Stu thought this was a unique way to highlight the importance of biochemical individuality, but Dr. Michael Colgan is anything but conventional.

Stu first became aware of Dr. Colgan's work whilst studying nutrition and reading his books on sports performance. Dr Colgan was an internationally acclaimed research scientist, author and lecturer who advised on nutrition and training to everyone from amateurs to Olympic world champions in numerous sports.

His fat feet statement was meant to be purposefully memorable in order to drive home a very important point: Biochemical individuality is vital to appreciate if you want to thrive in later life. Like our fingerprints, we are all biologically unique.

What this means is that when you apply changes in life to enhance your health or fitness, such as diet or exercise, you will always have to refine your methods so that they become as effective as possible.

Let's take your gut bacteria or microbiome as an example. We all know how important it is to have the right strains of beneficial bacteria in our gut and to limit the undesirable bacteria. Many people benefit from probiotic products, but what works wonders for one person might cause side effects like uncomfortable bloating or excess wind in another. You may need to experiment to find the one that works best for your system, either through trial and error or by getting a test to assess your current microbiome and identify the most suitable support.

This perfectly illustrates the importance of bio-individuality: just like fingerprints, your gut bacteria, and indeed your entire biology, are unique to you. The concept applies to every area of wellbeing. The more you embrace this, the easier it becomes to personalise your choices and genuinely support your health and vitality.

On the other hand, ignoring this principle and blindly following generalised health advice can lead to frustration, wasted effort or even worsening symptoms. You might feel like you're doing *all* the right things according to the latest trends – intermittent fasting, high-intensity workouts, specific supplements – yet still not feeling your best. In some cases, you may even be unknowingly aggravating underlying imbalances.

It's important to acknowledge that learning to tune into your unique needs can feel daunting at first. It might involve unlearning old habits, listening to your body in new ways or experimenting with approaches that feel unfamiliar or outside the mainstream. There may be moments of doubt or trial and error – and that's perfectly okay.

What matters most is developing a mindset of curiosity and compassion. Begin by noticing how your body responds to different foods, routines and environments. Keep a journal if it helps. Consider seeking support from a qualified practitioner who respects your individuality. And most importantly, trust that your body holds a great deal of wisdom. Your role is simply to listen and respond with care.

Over time, this personalised approach not only leads to better results, it also builds a sense of partnership with your body, replacing struggle with trust and confusion with clarity.

Knowing What's Right for You

A great foundation for personalising your approach to wellbeing is tapping into the wisdom of Ayurveda, a 5,000-year-old healing system from India. What's fascinating is that modern science is beginning to echo what Ayurveda has long understood: aligning with your natural constitution can have profound effects on your health. One study found that even a weeklong Ayurvedic-based retreat could shift patterns of gene expression linked to stress, inflammation and immune function.[3] Another discovered genetic markers that correspond with Ayurvedic mind-body types, offering a biological basis for the idea that we each have a unique constitutional blueprint.[4] In other words, the principles of Ayurveda are not only timeless, they're increasingly being validated by contemporary research.

The literal meaning of Ayurveda is the science of life:

    Ayus = Life

    Veda = Knowledge/Science.

Ayurveda provides practical tools for leading a long, healthy and happy life. There is no "one size fits all" prescription for wellbeing. Ayurveda embraces our individuality by recognising that each of us is made up of three core energies, or doshas: Vata, Pitta and Kapha. A dosha is like an inner blueprint, a unique blend of physical, mental and emotional traits that influences how you feel, think and thrive. Everyone has all three doshas within them, but usually one or two are dominant. Understanding your dosha can help you make more personalised choices in food, exercise routines and even emotional wellbeing, so you can stay in balance and feel your best as you get older.

To help visualise these types, it can be helpful to compare them to the Western concept of the three body types: ectomorph, mesomorph and endomorph. These describe different physical builds that you may have come across in fitness or sports science. They align closely with the Ayurvedic doshas, offering a familiar way to understand your unique constitution.

Vata and Ectomorph

Vata types align closely with the ectomorph body type. Just like ectomorphs, Vata individuals are typically lean, with light frames and smaller bone structures. They often have a slender, delicate build, with fast metabolisms and sometimes struggle to gain weight or muscle easily.

Pitta and Mesomorph

Pitta types resemble the mesomorph body type, known for their natural muscularity, medium build and athletic prowess. Pitta individuals, like mesomorphs, have a balanced bone structure and often experience good muscle tone and endurance. They tend to have robust metabolisms, gaining and losing weight relatively easily.

Kapha and Endomorph

Kapha types correspond well with the endomorph body type. Endomorphs, like Kaphas, have larger, broader frames, often with a naturally soft, round appearance. They tend to have a slower metabolism and are more prone to weight gain, especially as they age. Kapha types and endomorphs both exhibit resilience, steadiness and a tendency toward physical strength.

Tailoring Your Approach to Wellbeing

Some people prefer to focus on dietary and exercise strategies tailored to their body type. We have found that the Ayurvedic emphasis on individual constitution provides a more personalised approach to wellbeing strategies. The three doshas combine differently in every person, meaning that while we all have aspects of each dosha, most people are guided by a primary or a blend of two dominant doshas, known as a bi-doshic constitution. This unique combination shapes not only how we respond to the world but also how we experience ageing.

Vata-Pitta

What to Expect:

>**Body and mind**: Vata-Pitta types often experience a blend of high energy and creativity (from Vata) with a sharp focus and drive (from Pitta). As they age, they may notice an increase in physical dryness (from Vata) or occasional inflammation (from Pitta). This combination can sometimes lead to anxiety, sleep disturbances and digestive sensitivities, especially when Vata energy increases with age.

>**Common challenges**: Joint pain, dry skin, digestive upset, irritability and occasional burnout.

Balancing Tips:

>**Diet**: Emphasise warm, nourishing foods that aren't too spicy, such as cooked vegetables, grains and soups with healthy fats like ghee.

Routine: Regular routines are key; try to wake up, eat and sleep at the same times each day. Incorporate relaxation practices like gentle yoga and meditation.

Mindful cooling: Since both doshas are prone to overstimulation, it's important to balance activity with regular moments of rest and cool-down periods, especially in warmer months.

Pitta-Kapha

What to Expect:

Body and mind: Pitta-Kapha types often have a strong constitution, a steady mind and natural resilience. They tend to maintain muscle tone and physical strength well as they age. However, they may be prone to stubbornness, overcommitment or even complacency if routines are too repetitive. Ageing may bring concerns with weight gain (from Kapha) or inflammation (from Pitta), especially if lifestyle habits become too sedentary.

Common challenges: Weight management, sluggish digestion, skin sensitivity and irritability.

Balancing Tips:

Diet: Focus on light, fresh foods with lots of vegetables and fruits. Avoid heavy or overly oily foods that could weigh you down.

Routine: Regular exercise, ideally in the morning, can keep both doshas balanced. Engage in a mix of aerobic and resistance activities to maintain muscle tone and reduce excess Kapha energy.

Mental variety: Pitta-Kapha types benefit from mental stimulation and social engagement. Hobbies, creative projects and time with friends can keep both mind and body active.

Vata-Kapha

What to Expect:

Body and mind: This dosha combination blends the lightness and creativity of Vata with the steadiness of Kapha, resulting in an adaptable yet grounded personality. As Vata energy rises with age, people with a Vata-Kapha constitution may struggle with physical stiffness (from Kapha) and mental restlessness (from Vata). Ageing may bring slower digestion, occasional fatigue and a tendency to feel unmotivated or disconnected.

Common challenges: Joint stiffness, fatigue, occasional anxiety, weight gain and feeling "stuck" in routines.

Balancing Tips:

Diet: Incorporate warming, easy-to-digest foods and limit heavy or overly cold foods. Spices like ginger and cinnamon can help stimulate digestion.

Routine: Set up consistent times for meals, exercise and rest to avoid feeling scattered. Gentle stretching or yoga can relieve stiffness.

Gentle invigoration: To avoid stagnation, add a little variety to your day. Small changes, like trying new recipes or taking different routes for a walk, can keep your mind engaged without overwhelming your Kapha side.

Identifying your mind and body type or dosha allows you to adapt your diet, routines and lifestyle choices to align with your natural tendencies. In turn, this enables you to find balance and boost your vitality as you age.

You can find a Mind/Body Type Quiz on our website www.getstrongfitandhappy.com.

Learning the Hard Way

Like many people, Sue was intrigued by the compelling science behind intermittent fasting, the keto diet and cold showers. She got excited about the prospect of more energy, sharper mental focus and losing weight. So she threw herself into it. She skipped breakfast and fasted until midday. She swapped comforting meals for high-fat, low-carb dishes. She started each morning with a brisk cold shower, determined to become one of those energised, glowing people she'd seen in the health magazines.

At first, she was highly motivated. But it didn't take long before she started feeling…off. She wasn't losing weight – she was gaining it. She felt sluggish, not sharp. Her digestion became heavy, her energy dipped and instead of feeling energised and proud after a cold shower as so many other people had said, she just felt cold and a little defeated. It was frustrating. She was doing "all the right things." Or so she thought.

It wasn't until she revisited what she'd learned about Ayurveda and her Kapha constitution that things began to make sense. Kapha types naturally have a slower metabolism. Cold, heavy, oily foods and activities that reinforce stillness or dampness, like skipping breakfast, consuming lots of fats or taking cold showers, can aggravate those tendencies rather than help them.

Once Sue made changes that suited her Kapha nature, like eating a light, warming breakfast, favouring energising spices and lighter meals, sticking to regular routines and swapping cold showers for invigorating walks, Sue felt more energised and centred again. That experience reminded Sue how easy it is to be swayed by mainstream advice, even when it's backed by science. The most transformative lesson from this was not from following a trend, but from listening to her body and honouring her individual nature.

Actively listen to your body, tune into its messages. Your body constantly talks to you, and it is so important that you learn to develop the ability to interpret what it is telling you. It responds to different stimuli all the time, which can manifest in many different ways; pain or discomfort being one of the most common. Rather than looking for the cause, we often just reach for the painkillers, which is basically telling our body to shut up! If you can develop the skill of listening to your body and tuning into its subtle messages, you'll be better able to nip issues in the bud. Don't ignore rashes, fatigue, digestive upsets, brain fog or poor sleep, for example. Instead, use these messages to get to the root cause of the issue.

The point we want to make here is that you should always question anything out of the ordinary, and then either monitor or act. That doesn't mean to say you have to become a hypochondriac, only that you should have your own inbuilt radar that picks up on signs and symptoms as soon as they occur. This skill is something that needs to be mindfully practised until it becomes habitual. Ayurvedic practices can help here. Unfortunately, many people in our revved-up, fast-paced society wait until their body shouts and screams at them before taking action. It can then take so much longer to heal. We've both been guilty of that.

Listening to your body is also crucial when it comes to exercise. Stu has seen too many people continue to train on what is obviously the start of an injury, instead of stopping and catching it before it develops into something more serious.

Tuning Into Your Body's Inner Wisdom

While having goals for our health and vitality can guide and motivate us, sometimes those targets end up distracting us from what truly matters. Some people we have worked with almost obsessively count the number of days they have exercised and will not miss a day, even when they start to experience problems; the urge to train runs roughshod over any compassion they might have for their body. The result is almost always the same: spending weeks or even months nursing a chronic or acute injury, or in more extreme cases, surgery.

One of the most powerful aspects of knowing yourself is learning how to tune into your body's messages. Like many others, we've often ignored the early signs, waiting until our bodies shouted through pain or exhaustion instead of responding to the quieter signals that came first. Had we noticed those subtler cues, we may have resolved things with far less effort and disruption.

Your body is constantly communicating – through subtle shifts in energy, mood, digestion, sleep and even intuition. When we learn to listen, this awareness becomes one of our greatest guides to vitality and balance.

In recent years, we've seen an explosion in health-monitoring technology, from fitness watches to sleep trackers and apps that analyse everything from steps to stress levels. They provide data that our grandparents could have only dreamed of! These tools can be helpful for gathering information, but there's a risk: the more we rely on external devices to tell us how we're doing, the more we can drown out our body's voice.

When we outsource our self-awareness to a screen, we may start to ignore the quieter signals within, those early whispers of imbalance that technology can't always detect. And in some cases, people become so preoccupied with daily data that they overlook how they actually feel. For example, in the drive to hit a 10,000-step daily goal on their app, they ignore their tiredness and their body's need for rest, which could lead to exhaustion rather than vitality. Over time, this disconnection can leave you feeling out of sync with yourself, less confident in your own intuition.

Technology can be a helpful guide, though we feel it needs to be a complement rather than a replacement for your own embodied wisdom. True wellbeing comes from knowing yourself from the inside out. It can take time to acquire this skill, but it's worth the effort for your long-term health.

Final Thoughts

The journey of ageing is not about becoming someone different; it's about returning to who you've always been at your core. As we shed outdated roles, external expectations and one-size-fits-all trends, we create space to reconnect with the deeper wisdom that's been within us all along. Knowing yourself means tuning in, not just to your thoughts or your emotions, but to your body's messages, your values, your unique needs and your inner truth. And it's never too late to start.

By honouring your individuality, whether through understanding your Ayurvedic type, questioning the labels you've absorbed, listening more deeply to your body or choosing wellness strategies that truly fit, you empower yourself to live a life that feels aligned, fulfilling and free.

You are not defined by the years behind you but by the choices you make today. Embrace this moment to live as the person you were always meant to be. Take a moment today to listen to your body or question a label. Knowing yourself is the key to a life that feels authentic, vibrant and uniquely yours.

This grounded sense of knowing who you truly are also provides an inner resilience for dealing with life's inevitable ups and downs. In the next chapter, we'll explore how to draw on that clarity and strength when facing the challenges that ageing can bring.

> *"At the centre of your being, you have the answer; you know who you are and you know what you want."*
>
> *– Lao Tzu*

CHAPTER 5
Navigating Life's Challenges

"Challenges are what make life interesting. Overcoming them is what makes life meaningful."

– Joshua J. Marine

Keeping a positive approach to getting older will always be tested by life's inevitable challenges. As we move through the second half of life, the challenges we encounter shift from the familiar busyness of building a career or raising a family to navigating completely new challenges, unique to this stage of life: adapting to the retirement that redefines our sense of purpose, the loss of loved ones, the unexpected pressure that accompanies supporting elderly parents and more.

The realisation that we're attending more funerals than weddings could be seen as one of life's rites of passage. Do you have a particular funeral you remember that felt like a turning point in your perception of the time you have left? Perhaps it was the first funeral of a school friend or a close relative who had been a valued mentor, someone you'd imagined would always be around.

Each funeral attended can act as an unwanted yet sometimes necessary reminder of the finite nature of life and our own mortality. Each will have a different impact, from the memories, thoughts and feelings it ignites, to dealing with the loss of that person in our lives and adapting to the world without them in it. These moments can feel destabilising and overwhelming.

There are also the more familiar challenges that take on a newer meaning at this stage of life. For example, losing your job following a restructure at work has become the norm in the 21st century. Many of us have become used to reinventing ourselves to adapt to the continually changing job market. However, when we experience this in the later stages of our career, different concerns arise: from the relevance of our skills, expertise and experience in the ever-faster changing world of work to fears around competing for roles with far younger candidates.

That's why we feel this chapter really matters. How we meet life's inevitable challenges directly impacts *how* we age. Not just physically, but psychologically and emotionally. Facing challenges with intention – rather than avoidance, burnout or resignation – increases our self-awareness, deepens our inner resilience, builds our sense of perspective and helps us be more resourceful and adaptable.

You may be reading this chapter wondering: *Do I really need another pep talk about how challenges are secretly blessings in disguise?* It's a valid reaction. When we're in the thick of something hard, being told to "look for the opportunity" often feels dismissive and damn right annoying! More often than not, challenges don't feel like growth opportunities at the time; they feel isolating, disheartening and sometimes all-consuming.

That said, without challenges, we stagnate. Whether big or small, they divert our attention away from our goals and give us a chance to take stock and reflect. Like mistakes, setbacks and tough challenges often provide our greatest opportunities to learn and develop. As Judi Dench's character says in the film *The Best Exotic Marigold Hotel*, "The only real failure is the failure to try. And the measure of success is how we cope with disappointment."

In the river of life, its twists and turns can deepen our appreciation for what we already have – and sometimes carry us in a completely new direction, one that proves far more fulfilling than if we'd clung to the branch at the bend, resisting the flow.

We often get well-meaning advice suggesting that all we need to do is "think positively," "look on the bright side" or "stay strong" when life gets hard. Phrases like "everything happens for a reason," "it is what it is" or "time heals all wounds" are often offered with good intentions, but they can leave us feeling unseen, especially when we're in the middle of something deeply painful or uncertain.

Instead of glossing over the discomfort, this chapter provides a grounded, holistic and realistic approach to navigate and master the typical challenges that this period of our life brings. We know full well that when you're going through a tough time, it's not possible or helpful to search for the silver lining. Instead, we focus on building emotional flexibility, self-compassion and practical strategies to help you navigate life's inevitable challenges.

Reframing Thoughts and Feelings

Life's challenges often stir up a cascade of emotions: fear, frustration, sadness or self-doubt. These reactions are completely natural, rooted in our evolutionary need to protect ourselves from perceived danger or uncertainty. But if we leave these thought patterns unexamined, they can keep us stuck, amplifying stress and draining our resilience over time.

When we had to find a way to pay for the expensive care-home fees of Stu's mum, we made the difficult decision to sell her home. The process was anything but smooth. The sale fell through not once, but three times. Each time, hope would rise – only to be dashed again.

After a fourth buyer came along, we thought we were finally through the worst. A completion date was set for the first week of the year, and we allowed ourselves to look forward to the year ahead. *This year was going to be different*, we told ourselves. Then, the day before completion, the buyer pulled out. We remember the sinking feeling in our stomachs, the swirl of thoughts: *Will this ever end? What if we can't afford her care? Why does this keep happening? What are we doing wrong?*

This was not the way to start the new year. Realising that we needed to focus on what we could control, we tuned into our inner dialogue and recognised the pattern of powerlessness and hopelessness. With conscious effort, we chose to shift those thoughts. We reminded ourselves that we'd find a way through, because we always had.

We turned to Bach Flower Remedies, which offer gentle, natural support for restoring emotional balance. Developed in the 1930s by Dr. Edward Bach, a British physician and bacteriologist, the remedies were born from his deep concern for the emotional wellbeing of patients, particularly influenced by his experiences caring for injured soldiers during the First World War. He came to believe that unresolved emotional distress often lay at the heart of physical illness. Drawing on his medical training and intuition, he created a system of remedies using wildflowers and plants, each designed to help ease specific emotional states, like fear, overwhelm or despair.

Dr. Bach saw them as an emotional first aid kit, something accessible and practical for people to use whenever they needed to feel centred again.

Can you believe that even though Sue is a Bach Flower Remedy Practitioner, she didn't initially use them during this challenging time? She was immersed in *"What's the point?"* mode. That alone should have been the sign that she needed gorse!

Eventually, we did reach for the plant-based remedies: gorse for hopelessness, Rescue Remedy for the immediate emotional stress, and elm for feeling overwhelmed by all the responsibility. These small drops, along with consciously choosing to think more positively, became an anchor through that tough time.

The house did eventually sell. But more importantly, we learnt the importance of tuning into our inner dialogue, noticing what we were feeling inside and choosing more empowering self-talk.

Seven Typical Thoughts and Feelings

Outlined below are seven typical reactions when encountering demanding challenges and ideas to reframe and replace them. Consciously choosing different thoughts and feelings can be tough when we're immersed in a challenge, and so suggestions of Bach Flower Remedies have been included. Think of them as an emotional first aid kit. A couple of drops in a glass of water or a cup of tea will bring back balance and harmony.

1. *"I can't handle this."*

Typical feeling: Overwhelm, fear or helplessness.

Why it happens: New or unexpected challenges can make us feel unprepared or unequipped to cope, triggering a fight-or-flight response.

Shift to a new thought: "I've faced difficulties before, and I have the strength to face this too."

Suggestions:

- Review past challenges you've overcome. List the qualities you demonstrated, for example, patience, resourcefulness, creativity, methodical etc. Reflect on how you can apply those same qualities now.

- Think of someone who has dealt with a similar issue and may be able to share insights and ideas.

- Break the problem into smaller, manageable steps. Taking even one small action can reduce feelings of helplessness.

Bach flower remedy: Elm

Emotion before remedy: Feeling overwhelmed and doubting your ability to cope with responsibilities.

What to expect from the remedy: A renewed sense of confidence, capable of handling tasks calmly and effectively.

2. *"This will never get better."*

Typical feeling: Hopelessness, despair or impatience.

Why it happens: We tend to catastrophise when faced with uncertainty, imagining the worst-case scenario.

Shift to a new thought: "This is temporary, and I'm taking steps to improve it."

Suggestions:

- Practise mindfulness to stay present and avoid spiralling into "what if" scenarios.
- Keep a journal to track progress. Writing down one small improvement you notice each day, no matter how minor, can reinforce the belief that things will get better.

Bach flower remedy: Gorse

Emotion before remedy: Hopelessness and a belief that nothing will improve.

What to expect from the remedy: A renewed sense of hope and belief in the possibility of positive change.

3. *"I'm not strong enough for this."*

Typical feeling: Inadequacy, fear of failure or self-doubt.

Why it happens: Challenges can confront us and due to our perceived limitations, we question our ability to cope.

Shift to a new thought: "I am stronger than I think, and I can learn as I go."

Suggestions:

- Use affirmations to reinforce your inner strength: "I am capable. I am resilient."

- Seek support from loved ones, mentors or support groups. Sometimes, strength lies in asking for help.

- Stand in front of a mirror daily and say affirmations, such as "I am learning," or "I trust myself to find a way forward."

Bach flower remedy: Larch

Emotion before remedy: A lack of self-confidence and fear of failure.

What to expect from the remedy: A belief in your abilities and the courage to take risks.

4. *"Why me?"*

Typical feeling: Anger, resentment or self-pity.

Why it happens: When life feels unfair, it's easy to dwell on the seeming injustice of your situation.

Shift to a new thought: "This is happening, so what can I do about it? How can I grow from it?"

Suggestions:

- Reframe the challenge as an opportunity to learn.
- Write down three positive outcomes that could arise from the challenge, even if they are lessons or new perspectives.
- Keep a gratitude journal to counter feelings of unfairness. Recognising what is still good in your life can balance feelings of resentment.

Bach flower remedy: Willow

Emotion before remedy: Resentment, self-pity and a sense of unfairness.

What to expect from the remedy: A renewed ability to take responsibility for your perspective and find peace in the situation.

5. *"I'm stuck."*

Typical feeling: Frustration, inertia or hopelessness.

Why it happens: When solutions aren't immediately apparent, we may feel paralysed or unable to move forward.

Shift to a new thought: "I'm exploring new ways to move forward."

Suggestions:

- Write down as many possible actions as you can think of, no matter how small or unconventional. Pick one to try today.

- Brainstorm ideal scenarios and possible solutions. Often, simply listing options can reveal a way forward.

- Try something new, even if it's unrelated to the challenge. A fresh perspective often emerges from new experiences.

Bach flower remedy: Hornbeam

Emotion before remedy: Feeling mentally and physically fatigued, lacking motivation.

What to expect from the remedy: A renewed sense of energy and the ability to take action.

6. *"I'm alone in this."*

Typical feeling: Isolation, sadness or discouragement.

Why it happens: Challenges can feel uniquely personal, making it hard to see that others may have faced similar struggles.

Shift to a new thought: "I am not alone, and I can connect with others who understand."

Suggestions:

- Speak to an empathic and supportive friend. An informal chat, asking them to listen and letting them know that there's no need for them to offer solutions, can be immensely freeing. Sometimes, just putting your thoughts into spoken words can help to trigger ideas that you otherwise would not have considered.

- Reach out to a support group, community or online forum where people with similar experiences share their stories. Choose carefully – you want to avoid groups where the focus is on keeping stuck in the problem!

- Foster connections so you can create a strong sense of belonging and remind yourself of the joy that comes from shared experiences. Organise get-togethers with friends and family, even if it's just meeting up for a quick coffee. Look for reasons to celebrate life and make time for meaningful conversations with loved ones. Prioritise joining a club or taking classes where you can meet like-minded people. Commit to contacting at least one person today.

- Seek out books, podcasts or articles that provide inspiration and remind you of your shared humanity and give you a sense of connection.

Bach flower remedy: Heather

Emotion before remedy: A sense of isolation and self-absorption in your struggles.

What to expect from the remedy: The ability to connect with others and find comfort in shared experiences.

7. *"This shouldn't be happening."*

Typical feeling: Denial, frustration or resistance.

Why it happens: We often resist changes that disrupt our sense of control or stability.

Shift to a new thought: "This is happening, and I can adapt to it."

Suggestions:

- Practise radical acceptance. This doesn't mean giving up; rather, it is acknowledging the reality of the situation so you can focus on actionable steps forward. Spend five minutes reflecting on one aspect of the challenge you can't change. Then identify one thing you can control and commit to acting on it.

- Engage in activities that help ground you, such as yoga, meditation or spending time in nature.

Bach flower remedy: Rock water

Emotion before remedy: Rigid expectations and resistance to change.

What to expect from the remedy: Flexibility and acceptance of life's natural flow.

When Life Doesn't Go to Plan

> *"Option A is not available.*
> *So let's just kick the shit out of Option B."*
>
> – Sheryl Sandberg

This quote comes from Sandberg's book *Option B: Facing Adversity, Building Resilience, and Finding Joy,* which she co-wrote with psychologist Adam Grant. She used it to describe how she moved forward after the sudden death of her husband, acknowledging that life doesn't always go to plan, but we can still live fully in the version of life we now face.

When we carry a vision in our minds of how life *should* look, it can feel like a profound shock when that version is no longer possible. Option A might have been a particular career path, good health, a long future with someone we love or simply the life we imagined for ourselves or someone close to us. When that path is taken from us, we're faced with a choice: Resist reality and remain stuck in pain or find the strength to embrace a different version of life – Option B – and live it as fully as we can.

Sue had to learn this lesson the hard way. In her heart, Option A meant her hardworking mum enjoying a well-earned, idyllic retirement, finally free to indulge in hobbies she hadn't had time for before, living in the treasured family home that had been the heart of their lives for fifty years. Her mum, vehemently independent, had always insisted she would never leave her home.

Then came a series of health challenges, including dementia. Remaining at home was no longer safe or sustainable. And so, despite her wishes, Sue's mum had to move into a care home. Even though the care home was like a plush hotel, full of caring staff and a wonderful place to live, every time Sue visited her mum, she'd leave with a heavy heart. It wasn't *supposed* to be this way. Her mum deserved more, she thought. Sue found herself grieving not only the progression of the illness, but the loss of the life she had imagined her mum would have.

It was only when she realised that she needed to let go of what *should* have been, and started accepting what *was*, that she could be more present and less emotionally drained after each visit. She realised that while she couldn't change the situation, she *could* change how she related to it.

That's why we developed the 3-A Framework: to help people get unstuck, find a sense of calm amidst disruption and take meaningful steps forward. Sue applied this simple but powerful approach to help her cope with her mum's dementia. This has transformed her mindset and enabled her to ensure every visit with her mum is cherished and special. We hope it will be equally as useful to you to navigate whatever Option B you may be facing.

The 3-A Framework:
A Guide to Navigating Life's Challenges

When challenges arise, it's easy to feel overwhelmed, stuck or unsure of how to move forward. Whether you're facing a loss, a life transition or an unexpected health concern, your first response might be confusion, resistance or even numbness. That's entirely human.

But staying in that place for too long – looping through the same thoughts, avoiding decisions or denying what's happening – can leave you drained, disconnected and emotionally exhausted.

The 3-A Framework – Acknowledge, Accept, Adapt – is a simple, practical way to help you move through difficult moments. It doesn't try to sugar-coat the hard stuff. It just gives you a way to meet it with more calmness, clarity and composure.

Following this framework enables you to replace that common dispiriting feeling of life happening *to* you. You're giving yourself the space to pause, get honest about what's really going on and respond in a way that supports you not just in the moment, but for the longer term. It can help you gain more clarity, feel more focused and respond rather than react. It's a simple way to move from resistance to resilience.

When people don't have a process like this, they often stay stuck, caught in a loop of "Why is this happening?" or "This isn't how it was supposed to be." We can find ourselves denying reality, pretending we're fine when we're not, feeling sorry for ourselves or trying to push forward without having really processed what's happening. This can lead to drawn-out stress and even burnout.

When you take the time to acknowledge what's happening, accept your thoughts and feelings with compassion, and then consciously choose how to adapt, you free yourself. You become more resourceful, more centred and more connected to your own inner strength.

Step 1: Acknowledge – See the Situation Clearly

Recognise the challenge without denial or resistance. By naming the problem and your emotions, you bring it into focus.

Key questions to ask:

- What is happening right now?
- What are the facts versus assumptions or fears?
- What's within my control, and what isn't?

Mindset shift: "I see this challenge clearly, and I am ready to face it."

Exercises

> **Name it to tame it:** Write down the challenge and your emotions. Use simple, objective language e.g. "I lost my job, and I feel anxious about what's next."
>
> **What's really happening?** Spend a few minutes distinguishing between facts (what is true) and fears (what you're imagining).

Step 2: Accept – Embrace Your Reaction with Curiosity

Allow your emotions and thoughts to surface without judgement. Acceptance doesn't mean you like the situation; it means you make space for it.

Key questions to ask:

>How am I feeling about this challenge?

>What message might my emotions be trying to communicate?

>How can I be kind to myself in this moment?

Mindset shift: "It's okay to feel this way right now."

Exercises

>**Curious observer mindset:** Spend five minutes labelling your emotions, e.g. "This is frustration." Visualise these feelings as clouds passing by.

>**Journaling prompts for acceptance:** Reflect on your emotions: "What am I feeling? Why might I be feeling this way? How can I treat myself with compassion?"

Step 3: Adapt – Choose a New Way Forward

Move from reaction to action. Identify one small, constructive step to address the challenge. This step restores your sense of control and momentum.

Key questions to ask:

What is one small step I can take today?

How can I reframe limiting beliefs into empowering ones?

What have I learned from this challenge?

Mindset shift: "I am capable of finding solutions and moving forward."

Exercises

One small step plan: Identify and commit to one manageable action, such as researching support groups in your area.

Reframe to reclaim: Write down a limiting belief, like "I can't do this," and reframe it into an empowering one, "I can learn and grow through this."

Typical Challenges

"In the middle of difficulty lies opportunity."

– Albert Einstein

Outlined below are typical challenges that many of us find as we navigate this stage of life. When dealing with these challenges, it's easy to feel you're on your own. We hope this section helps you feel less isolated, reframes the challenge and gives you practical things you could do. Since time is often tight when immersed in challenges, we've also included some suggestions based on the time you have available.

Health Issues

The challenge: Coping with chronic conditions, fear of decline and the mental toll of ongoing health challenges.

The opportunity: Health challenges can serve as a wake-up call to slow down, prioritise self-care and reconnect with what truly matters.

To-Do List Ideas

Maintain faith in your body's capacity to heal: Focus on what your body can do, rather than what it can't.

Holistic wellness: Explore new forms of exercise, nutrition or mindfulness practices that support healing.

Gratitude for the present: Use health challenges as a reminder to cherish each day and celebrate small victories.

Research latest medical advances: Amazing discoveries are being made all the time to prevent and cure health conditions, so it's always worth researching the latest advancements. In the Resources section of our website, www.getstrongfitandhappy.com, you'll find recent studies showing medical advancements in illnesses often associated with getting older, including suggestions of things you can do to support your body.

If You've Got a Moment

5 minutes: Take three deep breaths, focusing on gratitude for your body's current abilities.

10 minutes: Write down one positive habit you'd like to adopt this week, such as drinking more water or stretching daily.

30 minutes: Try a new wellness practice, such as yoga, tai chi or a guided meditation.

Caring for Elderly Relatives

The challenge: Balancing the emotional and practical demands of caregiving with your own responsibilities and wellbeing. Life can feel on hold and it's easy to be fearful, wondering if this will be you in a few years' time. With so much of the focus on supporting your loved one, it is very easy to ignore your own needs. Constantly being in pink-alert or fight/flight mode and perhaps not sleeping well has, of course, a huge impact on your health. There'll be nothing left to give if your energy is depleted and your emotional tanks are empty.

The opportunity: Caregiving offers a unique chance to deepen your connection with your relative, honour their legacy and create lasting memories.

To-Do List Ideas

Legacy conversations: Use caregiving moments to ask about their life stories, advice and favourite memories. Capture these in a journal or audio recording.

Shared routines: Create simple rituals, like weekly movie nights or walks, to foster connection.

Reframe the role: When it feels like a burden, we have found it helpful to reframe it as an expression of love and gratitude for all they've done for you.

Nurture yourself: Just as we're reminded on an aeroplane to "put your own oxygen mask on first," caring for yourself isn't selfish, it's essential. As Peter Sage often says, "Give from your overflow." You'll be far more able to support your loved one if you've got plenty of energy and are feeling nurtured. It might be losing yourself in a favourite film, taking the afternoon off to meet up with a friend or any other small act that allows you a few moments to yourself

If You've Got a Moment

5 minutes:

Write down three things your loved one taught you that you want to pass on to future generations.

Step outside in the garden or walk to a park to reconnect with the present moment.

Splash water on your face. It's refreshing and also stimulates the vagus nerve, which helps calm the stress response.

Take 5 minutes to note down what's nurturing for you or a treat you can look forward to – taking the day off, going to the theatre, watching a film, reading a book, singing, dancing, drawing, cooking, gardening, etc., and keep the list handy. We know that when you're balancing multiple commitments and time is tight, doing anything for yourself can feel decadent. We've also learned how transformative doing something for yourself can be; it recharges your batteries and gives you a new lease on life.

10 minutes: Ask your loved one about their happiest childhood memory or what advice they'd give to their younger self. Listen to a favourite piece of music. Flick through a glossy magazine to switch off. Have a warm shower and visualise any unwanted emotions being rinsed away.

30 minutes: Record a video conversation with them to preserve their stories and wisdom. Curl up on the sofa with a favourite book that can transport you to a different time and place. Go for a walk in nature. Treat yourself to a drink from your favourite coffee shop and watch the world go by. Have a deep bath; feel the warm water relax your muscles, dissolve any tension and let go of any stresses from the day.

Selling the Family Home to Pay for Care

The challenge: Letting go of a home filled with cherished memories and navigating family dynamics around the decision.

The opportunity: This is a chance to honour the home's legacy while creating new opportunities for your loved one's care and comfort.

To Do List Ideas

Memory preservation: Take photos of meaningful spaces in the home and create a scrapbook or digital photo album. We've found that a digital photo frame in Sue's mum's room provides great triggers for conversation and special memories.

Family collaboration: Involve family members in sharing their favourite memories or choosing keepsakes.

A new chapter: From a practical perspective, selling the family home enables you to fund the care and support your loved one needs. It can also be seen as part of your loved one's legacy by providing another family with the opportunity to build their life and create their own treasured memories there.

If You've Got a Moment

5 minutes: Write a list of the happiest memories tied to the home.

10 minutes: Plan a farewell ritual, such as a family dinner where everyone shares their favourite story about the house. Choose a drawer, a shelf or a bedside table. Decluttering in 10-minute bite-sized chunks helps make the move less overwhelming.

30 minutes: Create a memory box with mementoes from the home for yourself or family members.

Moving a Parent Into a Care Home

The challenge: Navigating feelings of guilt, your parent's resistance and ensuring the care home meets their needs.

The opportunity: This transition is an opportunity to create a new sense of home for your parent while focusing on their care and comfort.

To-Do List Ideas

Advocacy role and assessing homes: Embrace the chance to ensure they receive the best possible care and attention. It takes time to research homes, but we've found that investing the time up front is worthwhile. Collate a list of parameters of what you're ideally looking for so you've got an objective way of assessing each home. Alongside attending a formal tour or open day, we found it useful to visit the care home unannounced, as you get a better feel of the atmosphere and the general morale of the staff.

Personalising the space: Help your parent decorate their new room with familiar items, such as family photos, a favourite chair or meaningful artwork.

Strengthening connection: Use this as a time to schedule regular visits or calls, building new traditions in their new setting.

If You've Got a Moment

5 minutes: Write down three things your parent loves that you can include in their new space. The Bach Flower Remedy Pine can be useful for managing any feelings of guilt. Walnut can be useful for your parent to help them adapt to this big life change.

10 minutes: Research activities offered by the care home and plan a visit to explore them. Put 10 minutes aside to locate and scan any paperwork, e.g., medication list, Power of Attorney, ID documents and save them all to a digital or place in a physical folder.

30 minutes: Create a full moving checklist – collate key tasks, medical records, packing, transportation, change of address notifications, emotional support prep. Having a plan calms the chaos.

Pack a "First Day Comfort Bag." Include luxury toiletries so they feel pampered, favourite snacks, magazines, anything that says, *"You are cared for."* Choose an outfit you know they feel great in so they arrive feeling good about themselves.

Before they move in, set up their room so it feels welcoming, familiar and homely. Add in a favourite cushion, mug, photo, pictures, soft blanket, treasured ornaments and coffee table books.

Facing Repeated "This is It" Moments

The challenge: Coping with the emotional whiplash of multiple "you'd better come" calls when a loved one's health falters, only for them to rally again. Each cannonball-to-the-stomach moment – anticipating a final goodbye that doesn't come – can leave you drained, anxious and stuck in a cycle of bracing for loss. Sue knows this all too well. Over the course of nine years, as her mum battled with sepsis and heart failure, Sue's family got seven calls. On each occasion, we'd rush to Mum's bedside, heart pounding, thinking, "This is it." We'd sit by her bed, holding her hand. Thankfully, she has pulled through each time, sometimes over a period of a few months, other times as quickly as a week. It brings a strange mix of emotions – the initial fear, followed by the relief, then the ongoing dread every time the phone rings.

The opportunity: These false alarms are a chance to build emotional strength, cherish the extra time with your loved one and shift from dread to presence, embracing an attitude that finds meaning in the now rather than fearing the inevitable.

To-Do List Ideas

Anchor in the moment: When the call comes, take a breath and focus on being fully present with your loved one, not just the outcome, seeing it as extra time to connect.

Release the cannonball: After each scare, let the tension out. This may be by talking it through with someone, going for a walk in nature to ground you or giving yourself permission to cry. We'd also recommend prioritising nurturing yourself as much as you can as the shock is emotionally exhausting.

Celebrate the rally: Mark their recovery, however small, with a quiet ritual – a shared cup of tea, flicking through a photo album or just a simple chat. This helps to reframe the experience as a gift, not just a reprieve.

If You've Got a Moment

5 minutes: Jot down three things you're grateful for about having your loved one around. Focus on these things the next time you're with them. It may be having the opportunity to give them a hug, chat about nothing in particular, remind them of a treasured memory, or simply have a cup of tea together.

The Bach Flower Rescue Remedy can help calm the immediate shock of a "this is it" call. There's always a bottle in Sue's bag! Mimulus can ease the lingering fear of what's next and Aspen is useful when you have that persistent apprehension.

10 minutes: After a scare, take a moment to reset. Step outside, breathe deeply and picture the cannonball dissolving into something lighter, like a feather. Write a quick note about what you enjoyed about being with them and what you're grateful for about the day.

30 minutes: Reflect on the ups and downs of their journey so far. Create a small "rally record" – a list or mental note of times they've pulled through – and use it to remind yourself of their resilience (and yours!) when the phone rings again.

Loss of a Loved One

The challenge: Grieving while managing practical responsibilities, navigating regret and supporting others in the family.

The opportunity: Grief can inspire reflection on life's fragility and the importance of honouring the legacy of those we've lost.

To-Do List Ideas

Legacy list: Create a document of your own preferences for eulogies, music and meaningful memories to ease the burden on others in the future.

Celebration of life: Plan annual rituals to celebrate your loved one's life, such as sharing stories, playing the music they loved or booking a table at their favourite restaurant.

Connection through sharing: Use the loss as an opportunity to reconnect with family and friends, reflecting on shared memories.

If You've Got a Moment

5 minutes: Light a candle and reflect on a favourite memory of your loved one.

Name three emotions you're feeling – "I feel numb, "I feel lost" or "I feel grateful." Grief is layered. Putting words to the feelings can help you stay connected to yourself and enable you to identify where you may need more support.

Send a text to a relative or friend who was also close to your loved one. Something as simple as "I'm thinking of you" can make a huge difference. You may want to share a brief memory, one of their typical phrases or something they laughed about. Checking in regularly via a quick call or a text is important. Consistency matters more than duration.

10 minutes: Find a favourite photo and put it in a frame.

Go for a short walk and talk to them in your mind. If they were here today, what would you say?

Sitting in a garden or in a park for 10 minutes can make a big difference. Being out in nature is inherently grounding and just a change of scene can help you see things in a new light.

30 minutes: Create a scrapbook, memory book or photo album to honour their life.

Write them a letter. Say what you miss, what you're struggling with, what you're grateful for. Writing can often release what words unsaid still carry.

Listen to a guided meditation for grief. This can be reassuring.

Cook one of their favourite meals for your family or friends. Food can be nurturing and nostalgic.

Traumatic Final Images of Loved Ones

The challenge: Overcoming the persistent, distressing memory of a loved one's pain or frailty in their final moments can overshadow their vibrant past and fuel fear of ageing or death.

The brain is wired to prioritise survival, and one way it does this is by latching onto emotionally intense experiences, especially those tied to pain, fear or loss. The brain's emotional alarm system flags these moments as critical for future reference, much like a built-in warning mechanism. When someone witnesses a loved one dying in pain or distress, that image gets etched into memory because it's loaded with emotional weight: grief, helplessness or even a subconscious fear of their own mortality. It's similar to why we vividly recall where we were during events like 9/11. The brain treats these moments as "high-alert" lessons, replaying them to prepare us for potential threats. Unfortunately, this protective mechanism can trap people in a cycle of replaying the distressing memories rather than the joyful ones, overshadowing the fuller, more vibrant story of a loved one's life.

Stu found it exceptionally hard to shake off the image of his mum's frail body in the hospital bed. It haunted him for months afterwards and dimmed the decades of memories of his vivacious and fun-loving mum. Stu longed for those images to be the first that came to his mind rather than the chilling hospital scene. Printing a favourite photo of his mum and putting it in a frame on his desk was a useful starting point as he saw it every day and it made him smile. Watching a video of his mum getting into hysterics when playing a game at Christmas also helped replace the harrowing image.

He then went on to collate an album of favourite shared memories, as suggested above.

Although time is the great healer when it comes to tough memories, Stu acknowledges now that he allowed that harrowing image to outstay its welcome. He wishes he'd thought about collating photos earlier and spent more time focusing on those happy memories.

The opportunity: This is a chance to reclaim the fuller story of your loved one's life, honouring their vitality and love. It's also an opportunity to consciously take your attention away from images that can contribute to a negative view of ageing.

To-Do List Ideas

Create a memory gallery: Visualise a mental space – a hallway or album – filled with joyful moments from your loved one's life and intentionally revisit these scenes to balance the painful ones.

Anchor the positive: Pair a happy memory with a physical object, such as a photo or keepsake, to ground you in their vibrancy whenever the distressing image surfaces.

Reframe with compassion: Acknowledge that the painful memory is not a fair reflection of their whole life. When you're ready, gently shift your focus to moments that reflect their essence. Think about how they'd like to be remembered and what images they'd like you to have in your mind when you think of them. This can take time, so be patient with yourself.

If You've Got a Moment

5 minutes: Write down three joyful memories of your loved one; specific moments that capture their spirit. It may be a night out, a special holiday, a trip to the seaside, how their eyes lit up when they talked about something they loved, the things that used to make them laugh, a quiet moment you shared together, their favourite cake, a spontaneous day out. The Bach flower remedy, Star of Bethlehem, can help soothe lingering shock or grief from those final images. Honeysuckle can assist in letting go of the past while cherishing the memories.

10 minutes: Pick one memory and replay it in your mind like a short film. What did they say, wear or do? Note sensory details such as the smell of their perfume, the colour of their outfit or the warmth of their smile to make it vivid.

30 minutes: Create a photo album of favourite images and special memories. In a notebook or journal, jot down treasured moments you shared, capture their catchphrases and idiosyncrasies. Then when the painful image creeps in, you can refocus on better times.

Final Thoughts

Later life comes with profound challenges, from losing loved ones, caring for elderly parents, retiring and redefining purpose to facing health concerns. These experiences can catch us off guard as they question the stories we've told ourselves about who we are and how life should unfold. They can also lead us to feel isolated and overwhelmed.

During the years we were working full-time while supporting ill parents, we found ourselves in constant trouble-shooter mode. Fire-fighting became the norm, tackling one issue at a time and finding quick fixes. It often felt like no sooner had we resolved one problem than another would appear, so there never seemed to be any time for ourselves, to reflect or to plan. Over the course of ten or more years, this became exhausting and impacted our health. What this taught us, though, was the importance of taking the time to pause, face up to the reality of the situation, regroup and get focused.

Our aim for this chapter is to remind you that you're not alone. We hope that some of the practical suggestions will help to bring fresh perspectives to the challenges you encounter, together with ideas for nurturing yourself. By recognising your natural responses, learning how to reframe difficult thoughts and drawing on resources that support your emotional wellbeing, you'll build strong foundations for dealing with whatever challenges life brings.

In the next chapter, we'll explore how life's challenges can often act as a catalyst for nudging us to seek deeper purpose and rediscover passions that bring clarity, joy and a renewed sense of direction at this stage of life.

"You can't stop the waves, but you can learn to surf."

– Jon Kabat-Zinn

CHAPTER 6
Purpose and Passion

"You know the Greeks didn't write obituaries. They only asked one question after a man died: 'Did he have passion?'"

– Marc Klein's *Serendipity* (film script)

Having a passion brings an extra spark to life. It provides purpose, focus and often an inner drive for mastery. It catalyses joy and can foster connections with others who share the same interest. Our passions often offer clues to the more elusive concept of our sense of purpose. Even when we're living it, purpose isn't always something we're consciously aware of. But clearly defining it can create a roadmap for living life with a profound sense of meaning.

Throughout life, we may feel an inner call to live more authentically and intentionally in order to feel truly fulfilled. That call often grows louder in the second half of life as we become more aware of life's finite nature and the roles we've played for many years begin to shift. For example, retiring from a career that once shaped you may lead to some questions about identity. It's at this point that living with purpose and passion becomes not just fulfilling, but essential. As one of Sue's coaching clients asked herself, "If not now, when?" When you're aligned with your purpose and fuelled by your passions, life becomes more vibrant and meaningful. You wake up with direction; decisions become clearer. You feel more alive. But even more profoundly, living this way meets all six of our core human needs – the drivers that shape our behaviour and give us a sense of wholeness.

Certainty. Purpose gives us a foundation, something solid we can stand on, even when life around us changes. It provides inner stability, reminding us who we are and what we stand for.

Uncertainty and Variety. By their very nature, our passions keep us interested in life and keen to find out more and look beyond the familiar. Our passions keep life exciting and engaging. It invites spontaneity, exploration and learning – an antidote to stagnation.

Significance. When we live our purpose, we are being true to ourselves. We matter, not in an ego-driven way, but in the sense that we know our life is making a difference. We feel seen, heard and valued, even if only by ourselves.

Love and Connection. When we're living in line with our purpose, we feel connected to our true self. By feeling more centred, we can connect with others more authentically, which can deepen relationships. Purpose can also involve connection with others, whether it's directly or through causes, connection with nature or something greater than ourselves.

Growth. Purpose-driven living naturally invites discovery. You evolve as you pursue what lights you up, constantly learning and becoming.

Contribution. Perhaps the most powerful of all: when we live in alignment with our purpose and passions, we give back. We contribute not just time or resources, but our unique essence: our presence, our perspective, our wisdom.

So, if you've ever asked yourself, *"Is there more to life than this?",* the answer is yes. And the map to that "more" is your purpose. Not something you need to chase or invent, but something you *uncover* by listening to what lights you up, energises you and connects you to something greater. What gives your life meaning? What lights you up inside, even when no one's watching? This chapter is about reigniting the inner spark that keeps us feeling vibrant and alive: our *purpose* and *passion*. These two forces are often what make the difference between simply existing and truly *living*, especially as we get older.

As we age, society sometimes nudges us toward winding down or stepping back – but the truth is, our later years can be the most purposeful and passionate of all. In fact, studies have shown that having a strong sense of purpose isn't just uplifting, it's good for our health. One study found that people with a clear sense of purpose lived longer, regardless of when they discovered it in life.[1] Another showed that living with meaning and direction contributes to better emotional wellbeing and overall health.[2] It's powerful evidence that finding purpose isn't just fulfilling, it's life-enhancing.

This chapter will explore how reconnecting with what truly matters to you can become a powerful antidote to the fear of ageing. Our purpose can sometimes be a quiet, intuitive whisper we haven't had time to pay much attention to. Even if you are already clear on your purpose, we hope this chapter will prove useful for reviewing it, refining it and perhaps even reigniting it!

PURPOSE AND PASSION

If you've ever thought, *"I'm too old to start something new"* or *"It's too late to discover what I'm here for,"* this chapter is here to challenge that thinking! You'll discover that purpose doesn't need to be grand or world-changing and passion doesn't need applause. Sometimes it's the often-unseen commitments – like painting in solitude, tending a garden or mentoring someone – that have the greatest impact.

We'll look at real-life examples of people who've embraced their later years with energy and intention, not because they had to, but because they *wanted* to. Their stories will inspire you to explore what lights you up or reignite something that's been long buried. We'll explore how purpose and passion can become your compass, not just to age well, but to *live fully*, no matter what age you are.

Living With Purpose and Passion

Living with purpose and passion isn't about seeking external validation; it's about honouring what makes you feel alive. Whether quietly or boldly, people who stay connected to what they love often radiate vitality.

Take Dame Judi Dench, for example. Despite age-related challenges like vision loss, she continues to grace the stage and screen with remarkable energy. Her enduring love for storytelling fuels her creativity and keeps her spirit vibrant.

Then there's Sir David Attenborough. Well into his 90s, he remains a powerful voice for the planet, passionately educating and advocating for the natural world. His sense of purpose hasn't waned. If anything, it's grown stronger with age.

And not all passions are lived in the spotlight. Eric Tucker, a self-taught painter, quietly created over 500 works capturing everyday life in Northern England. Though his art remained unseen during his lifetime, he painted purely for the joy of it. After his death, his work was discovered and celebrated; proof that passion doesn't need an audience to be meaningful.

Each of these individuals, in their own way, shows how purpose and passion can defy age, spark joy and leave a lasting legacy, with or without recognition.

Purpose Isn't Pious and Pompous

One of Sue's coaching clients, who was in her late fifties at the time, was at a crossroads after a restructure at work led to her leaving the company she had worked at since finishing school. She was searching for a new direction but struggling with the idea of "finding her purpose." The word itself felt pious and pompous to her, as if it required a grand mission or lofty calling. After reflecting on questions that enabled her to explore when she's at her happiest, how friends would describe her when she's at her best, the qualities she likes about herself, as well as her strengths and unique talents, she started to see that clarifying her purpose enabled her to live meaningfully and authentically.

Over time, she noticed there was a strong correlation between her sense of fulfilment and the extent to which she was living in line with the values, qualities and talents that comprise her sense of purpose. She called this her "North Star" – her personal compass. It wasn't a fixed destination or a job title, but a deep sense of inner clarity that helped guide her decisions and gave her life a renewed sense of direction and joy.

Purpose is Not Grandiose

> *"Beyond sculptures and symphonies, beyond great works and masterpieces is the greater, finer art of moulding a conscious life. Genius appears everywhere, but never so magnificently as in a life well lived."*
>
> – Karla McLaren

A well-lived life, as Karla McLaren suggests, isn't about achieving fame or creating world-renowned masterpieces. Instead, it's about living intentionally, shaping a life that reflects what's most important to you. What does a "life well-lived" mean to you? Have you ever paused to truly reflect on this?

John Lennon famously popularised the phrase, "Life is what happens to you while you're busy making other plans." It's a poignant reminder of how easy it is to become consumed by the demands of work, home, family and friends, leaving little time to consider whether we're living a life aligned with our deepest desires and aspirations. As we age and become more aware of life's finite nature, taking time to contemplate our purpose and what a well-lived life means becomes not just useful but essential. It's not just about achieving goals or pursuing hobbies; it's about aligning with what truly matters to you, living intentionally so life feels meaningful.

When you live with purpose, you feel energised and fulfilled. You gain clarity, strengthen your relationships and experience a renewed sense of vitality. Purpose-driven individuals often talk about serendipity and how unexpected opportunities flow into their lives. By following their "North Star", they feel they're being true to themselves and find that this also helps them create more lasting impacts on those around them.

The Importance of Purpose

Living with purpose is not just a "nice to have", it's essential for a fulfilled, healthy and vibrant life. In Chapter 3, we looked at the Six Human Needs and how lasting fulfilment comes when we consistently meet all of them in a balanced way. This is why having a purpose is so important: It allows you to meet each of these needs.

Without a sense of purpose, you might feel stuck in routines or disconnected from what truly matters. We've observed this in relatives and people we've worked with over the years. It shows up as a lack of motivation, a lack of clear direction or a vague sense that something's missing, even if life seems "fine" on the surface. Research backs this up. Studies show that a lack of purpose is linked to higher stress levels, increased risk of cognitive decline and poorer overall health.

Research published in *JAMA Network Open* found that purposeful living contributes to longevity and overall health in older adults.[3] One of the longest-running studies on happiness by Harvard University found that individuals with a clear sense of purpose reported higher levels of life satisfaction, which in turn impacted their physical health.[4] From a psychological perspective, studies show that purposeful activities trigger the brain's reward system, releasing hormones that enhance mood and motivation.[5] In regions where people frequently live to 100, such as Okinawa in Japan and Sardinia in Italy, having a purpose is considered a cornerstone of their longevity.[6]

Our Sense of Purpose Evolves Throughout Our Lives

"It's never too late to be what you might have been."

– George Eliot

Our purpose reflects our unique talents and innate qualities and aligns with our values. As we acquire new talents and interests throughout our lives, our purpose evolves over time. It's something to discover, rediscover, clarify and continuously cultivate.

You might believe that purpose is for the young, or that it's too late to find a meaningful path. Julia Child discovered her passion for cooking in her fifties and went on to revolutionise home cooking in America. As a schoolboy, Michael Palin remembers that, "the idea of travelling and exploring and adventure was very strong." He was in his mid-forties before embarking on his *Around the World in 80 Days* journey, which led to many other amazing trips across the globe and a new career as a documentary maker.

What aspirations or interests did you have as a child that you'd like to rediscover? Were you one of the fortunate individuals who knew exactly what they wanted from life and followed that path? At this point, these are just questions to ponder as you read this chapter.

Stu was a firefighter for 30 years, and whilst he enjoyed the work, particularly driving the fire appliances and the camaraderie, he never felt it was his true calling. He studied different career paths in an effort to achieve the success he was looking for. Ironically, he found his mission through being a Physical Training Instructor in the Fire Brigade. He found that the most fulfilling aspect of his work was sharing his knowledge as a Nutritionist and Personal Trainer to help his colleagues transform their health and fitness.

To build on his knowledge, Stu went to Canada in 2004 to train as one of Dr. Colgan's Certified Trainers in a specialist programme designed to improve muscular speed and strength in athletes – with principles that could be applied to anyone. Dr. Colgan was in his sixties at the time and performed strength exercises that most people forty years younger than him would struggle to do.

This was a true turning point for Stu; he realised that losing strength as you get older was not inevitable, as he had originally thought. Stu shared the principles and techniques he learned with his colleagues who needed to maintain a high level of fitness and muscular strength, whether they were in their twenties or their fifties. The sense of fulfilment he gained from helping his colleagues gave him an epiphany in the latter stage of his career and enabled him to finally discover his mission in life.

Without purpose, life can feel monotonous or aimless, leading to dissatisfaction or regret. Taking steps to discover your purpose allows you to live intentionally, connect deeply with others and leave a meaningful legacy.

When Sue was at infant school, like many children, she loved transporting herself to the imaginary world of the books she read or the stories that were read to her. Her favourite class was creative writing, where she could lose herself completely, not noticing the bell for playtime or that a sunny day had turned into a rainy day. Once she wrote a story and was sent to the Head Teacher's office.

She was terrified and automatically thought she was going to be told off for doing something wrong, but instead she was told that her story was enchanting and that one day she'd be a writer. As an adult looking back, the head teacher was probably simply being encouraging, but to her seven-year-old self, this exchange cemented the belief that she would be a writer when she grew up. She was so excited – this would be a dream come true. Then, as with many of us, her dream was placed on the back burner. Sue found at secondary school that she loved maths and science, so she learnt to be logical and rational. There was far less scope for nurturing an overactive imagination.

Although the idea of being a writer always felt part of her, there were so many reasons why she couldn't be – she didn't read enough, her vocabulary wasn't wide enough, she was no longer imaginative and then of course there was the comparison curse. What could she bring that would be different or of value to others?

One snowy morning in London, in a freezing cold office at a coaching supervision session, Sue's supervisor told her, "If you find yourself giving the same advice to your clients, you may want to ask if this is advice you need to take yourself." At the time, Sue was in her 12th year of being a career transition coach, helping people to explore their purpose and find roles that were truly fulfilling to them. She absolutely loved this work and felt she had found her true calling. However, she realised that she needed to take a bit of her own advice and dig a bit deeper beneath the surface to explore other ideas for her career and sense of fulfilment.

Exploring her sense of purpose in the same way as she did with her clients, that inner whisper of wanting to be a writer came to the surface. To begin with, all the reasons why she couldn't block her way forward. "Be realistic. This is for people who are far better with words than you," said a voice in her head. Then she took another bit of her own advice and reminded herself that it didn't matter what other people thought – just write because you enjoy it. If you've ever been put off starting something because you were concerned about whether you'd be good enough, just get into "sod it" mode and do it anyway. The enjoyment that comes from doing it is far more important.

Focus on What Truly Matters

In *Meditations for Mortals*, Oliver Burkeman reminds us that our time is finite, and we'll never accomplish everything we set out to do. Instead of striving for perfection or an unattainable level of productivity, he encourages us to embrace our limitations and focus on what truly matters. By accepting that we can't do it all, we free ourselves to invest our energy in what brings meaning and joy. Burkeman's philosophy reminds us that life's value isn't measured by how much we complete but by the depth of purpose and connection in what we choose to pursue.

For people who have a tendency to set the bar high for themselves, it's important to ensure they enjoy the journey rather than feel overwhelmed by the enormity of what they want to achieve. There will always be unfinished business and unachieved goals – the important thing is that you feel that inner sense of fulfilment and contentment.

This brings us on to the subject of bucket lists! We've never been fond of the term. It often feels like a checklist of arbitrary achievements - as if life would somehow be incomplete without ticking them all off.

And what then? Is there nothing else worth doing? Does finishing the list somehow grant permission to die? To us, if your list is fully completed, maybe it wasn't driven by a big enough sense of curiosity or adventure. Often, when people talk about their bucket lists, they mention the usual suspects – go-to goals that feel more like external influences than true inner callings.

So, as well as ticking off travel destinations or adrenaline-charged experiences, we invite you to tune inward as well. What stirs your soul? What makes you feel most alive, most yourself? If you like having a "bucket list," try also having a "soul list": a collection of experiences, contributions and connections that reflect your deepest values and longings. This could include things like learning a craft that fascinates you, mentoring someone who could benefit from your wisdom, expressing your creativity in a new way or immersing yourself in a cause that is very important to you. Ask yourself: "What do I want to experience, express or contribute in this lifetime, not to prove something, but to feel fully me?" By shifting the focus from external milestones to inner resonance, your journey becomes less about external expectations of achievement and more about inner alignment. That's where we feel purpose meets passion. where ageing becomes not a countdown but the opportunity to connect to a wider range of experiences that truly connect to what's most important to you.

Having Fun and Going With the Flow

Watching the film *Quartet* in 2012, the song "Are You Havin' Any Fun?" by Flanagan and Allen struck a chord with us. At the time, we were working very long hours trying to keep a business afloat whilst also working full-time on our day jobs. So, when Trevor Peacock and David Ryall sang the line "Are you havin' any fun? What are you getting out of living?" it made us realise that we'd got far too serious and busy working on a business that no longer gave us any joy. We knew the end product was of a high quality and it contributed to people's wellbeing, but we'd lost sight of enjoying the process.

It wasn't until we recognised that we were allowing a hardwired mindset of "if something is worth achieving, then it's got to be hard work" that we took stock and looked at ways we could make it easier and more enjoyable. Asking ourselves, *"Are we having any fun?"* we realised that fun was too small a part of our lives, something we felt we needed to earn. Automatically prioritising the to-do list and feeling guilty for having time off also added extra evidence that we'd got life out of balance. Reviewing what we love doing, what comes naturally to us and collating our innate values helped us to reevaluate what was important and helped us map out a new direction. So, the sense of purpose remained pretty much the same; it's just the way we went about achieving it was different.

Working towards achieving a sense of purpose should not create undue stress in your life. Some minor, manageable stress is fine, but if you are pursuing something that is ruining your life, you have to ask yourself, "What is the point of this?" Perhaps you need to redefine your purpose or find a different way to work towards it.

Ikigai

Ikigai is a Japanese concept that translates to "reason for being" and represents the intersection of what you love, what you're good at, what the world needs and what you can be rewarded for. Rooted in the philosophy of living with purpose and joy, ikigai emphasises balance and alignment between passion, skill and contribution. It's not about achieving perfection but about creating a meaningful and fulfilling life by engaging in activities that resonate with your inner self. By discovering your ikigai, you can uncover the unique purpose that drives you and transform it into a guiding compass for a vibrant and purposeful life. Ikigai is the sweet spot where your inner desires meet the external world's needs, creating a life that feels both joyful and purposeful.

> **The 4 Elements of Ikigai**
>
> 1. **What you love** (your passions)
>
> 2. **What you are good at** (your strengths)
>
> 3. **What the world needs** (your contributions)
>
> 4. **What you can be rewarded for** (financially or emotionally)

When someone close to us dies, that's often the time when we question what life is all about. After the loss of his wife, Michael Palin said, "A great sort of emptiness comes in." Reading that interview deeply resonated with Sue. It took her straight back to the raw early days of grief after her dad died – bent double in tears, wondering if life would ever be the same or feel okay again. There was a hollow ache that felt endless, an infinite black hole of sadness where even the simplest question, "What now?" felt impossible to answer. In those moments, it was hard to imagine feeling whole again or to see a way forward with any sense of purpose. But over time, there was a gradual, almost imperceptible shift, a deeper understanding of what truly mattered and what she wanted to assign her finite time to. The emptiness that

Michael Palin spoke of never truly gets filled again, but Sue has found that it provides a space for gaining clarity for living with greater intention, presence and meaning.

Rediscovering our Ikigai is key to turning our later years into some of the most meaningful and empowering of our lives. Ikigai, in many ways, combats the fear of ageing and helps us embrace the opportunities ahead with enthusiasm.

IKIGAI Framework

Many people approach purpose passively, waiting for it to "happen" or viewing it as elusive. We devised the IKIGAI Framework to help you actively uncover your purpose or help you redefine it to ensure it is relevant and true to this stage of your life. It's a step-by-step guide, making the abstract concept of purpose tangible and achievable.

I – Identify your passions

Purpose: Discover what excites and energises you.

Rediscovering what truly lights you up can feel surprisingly difficult, especially if you've spent years focused on caring for others, building a career or simply getting through life's demands. Many people find it hard to answer the question "What do I enjoy?" because their own passions have taken a back seat for so long.

You may feel out of touch with your own interests or worry that your passions aren't "worthy" or practical enough to pursue. That's completely normal. The key is to approach this step with curiosity, not pressure. Think of it as uncovering something that's been quietly waiting in the wings rather than inventing something new. Start by reflecting on moments in your life when you felt most alive, connected or deeply engaged. Don't limit yourself to big achievements. Look for everyday moments too. Ask yourself:

- Which activities absorb you so fully that you lose track of time and feel in the flow?
- What types of books, conversations or topics draw you in?
- What causes or issues stir something inside you?
- What did you love doing as a child or young adult, before life got busy?

If answers don't come right away, give it time. Try keeping a "passion journal" for a week. Jot down what energises or interests you, even in small ways.

Outcome: A clear understanding of your interests and passions.

K – Know your strengths

Purpose: Understand your natural talents and unique abilities.

- Note down and journal about compliments or feedback you frequently receive.
- If modesty gets in the way of acknowledging your strengths, write down a list of things you enjoy doing. There's a strong correlation between fulfilment and what we're good at. For example, if you enjoy detail-focused tasks, then your natural strengths may include thoroughness, diligence and setting high standards. If you get a sense of satisfaction from helping people,

then your strengths could include being thoughtful, supportive and caring. Please refer to the Further Resources chapter for ways to collate strengths.

- Reflect on challenges you've overcome and what they reveal about your strengths and abilities.

- Ask yourself:
    - What do others consistently say you're good at?
    - What comes easily to you that others struggle with?

Outcome: A list of core strengths and talents.

I - *Investigate your values*

Understanding what motivates and fulfils you is strongly linked to your values. We all have values, but we are often unconscious of them. Rather like DNA being the blueprint for our bodies, values provide the blueprint of who we truly are. We tend to notice them when they are not being honoured. For example, if openness is one of your values and you're working with colleagues with hidden agendas who don't share information, then you'll be demotivated. If you're reporting to a micromanager and autonomy is high on your list of values, then you'll feel out of kilter.

Purpose: Define the principles that guide your life and decisions.

- Select your top five values from the list included in the Companion Guide e.g. integrity, compassion, freedom.

- Reflect on moments of fulfilment and what values were present.

- Reflect on times when you did not feel centred. What values were being dishonoured?
- Ask yourself:
    - What principles guide your decisions and relationships?
    - What values feel non-negotiable to you?

Outcome: A defined set of personal values to anchor your purpose.

G – Gather inspirations

Purpose: Connect with role models and qualities that resonate with your aspirations.

- Create an "Inspiration Map" of people, stories or archetypes you admire.
- Ask yourself:
    - Who are your role models, and why?
    - What qualities or actions do they embody that inspire you?

Outcome: A deeper connection to qualities you aspire to emulate.

A – Align your mission

Purpose: Synthesise your passions, strengths, values and inspirations into a guiding statement.

- Use this formula:

- "I am [identity/passion], and I am here to [action] by leveraging [strengths] in alignment with [values]."

- Example:
  - "I am a storyteller, and I am here to inspire curiosity and connection by using my creativity and authenticity in alignment with my values of compassion and exploration."

Outcome: A personalised purpose statement.

I – Implement actions

Purpose: Transform your purpose into tangible, everyday practices.

- Identify small daily habits and long-term goals aligned with your mission.
- Ask yourself:
  - What's one small action I can take today to live my purpose?
  - How can I integrate my mission into my relationships and career?

Outcome: A clear action plan to live with purpose.

Final Thoughts

When you live with purpose, you feel energised and fulfilled. You gain clarity, strengthen your relationships and experience a renewed sense of vitality. Purpose-driven individuals often find unexpected opportunities, achieve a sense of invigorating personal growth and create lasting impacts on those around them. Purpose is uniquely personal and doesn't need to be world-changing. One of the most contented people we know is Sophia, a barista in our local coffee shop. She appears to make it her mission to brighten everyone's day through her warm welcome and engaging conversation. She always remembers the way the regulars prefer their coffee and goes out of her way to make every drink perfect. This is a great example of living with purpose. It's about finding meaning in what you do and the impact you can have on others, no matter how small it may seem.

If you need to discover or redefine your purpose, we hope the IKIGAI Framework is useful to you. It's not about achieving perfection but about aligning your life with what matters most. It's a journey of self-discovery, growth and contribution that can transform your later years into a time of vitality, meaning and joy. By taking these steps, you'll not only uncover your purpose but also create a legacy that inspires others. Purpose sets the direction, though it's what we do with it that defines us. The clarity that comes from knowing our purpose becomes truly powerful when it's lived, not just understood. In the next chapter, we explore how to turn insight into action and knowledge into a life fully lived. Purpose, like wisdom, only comes to life when it's embodied in our everyday choices.

> *"Growing older is no longer about compensating for lost or weakened capacities but rather about getting closer to embracing who we're meant to be. Each year that goes by connects us more to our purpose."*
>
> – Dr. Gladys McGarey

CHAPTER 7
Nothing Is Learned Until It Is Lived

"It is easy to overestimate the importance of one defining moment and underestimate the value of making small improvements on a daily basis."

– James Clear

We live in an age overflowing with information. We read books, watch documentaries, attend courses and scroll through endless advice online. And yet, how much of what we *know* do we actually *live*?

This chapter explores the vital shift from acquiring knowledge to embodying wisdom. It's about the transformation that happens when we stop passively collecting insights and start actively applying them through our choices, our relationships and our daily routines. In other words, it's not what we know that changes us – it's what we *live*.

From Knowing to Becoming

When we don't apply what we learn, the benefits stay theoretical. Research suggests that adults forget up to 75% of new information within just six days.[1] If we don't act on what we learn, we miss the opportunity to change our lives.

As we explored in the Life Wisdom, Know Thyself and Purpose and Passion chapters, we can benefit from the insights we have gained over the years, and focus on honouring what matters most to us so we can be true to ourselves. With the benefit of our experience, we can recognise what truly counts, spot patterns more clearly, and enjoy the freedom to realign our lives accordingly. In this chapter, we'll explore how we can consistently bridge the gap between learning and living so that knowledge becomes transformation, and wisdom becomes a way of being.

Best of Intentions

When Stu's dad died after a long and insufferable struggle, we vowed to be grateful for every day and not allow the stuff that doesn't matter in the greater scheme of things to get us down. This defining moment in our lives in 2005 gave way to a well-intentioned goal. Yet as life returned to some sort of normality, we soon lost that sense of perspective and returned to our old habits.

It wasn't until a friend of ours died six months later that we were reminded again of the futility of our ingrained habits of feeling stressed and worrying about the future. So, driving back from the funeral, we set ourselves the goal again of taking life in our stride, valuing every day and being in the moment. What we didn't know at the time was that our habitual behaviour is linked to our beliefs and ultimately who we are. We were focusing on the outcome rather than who we needed to be to approach life in the way we were aiming for.

So, however much we were committed to achieving the outcome, nothing was going to change for the long term, not without addressing our habitual thoughts and pre-programmed beliefs.

For example, if someone identifies as an anxious person, it's likely that their thoughts are fear-based, which heavily impacts their behaviour. They may worry too much, focus on the worst possible scenario and stay within their comfort zone as they're concerned about the uncertainty of the future. Thinking differently will help them move towards their goal, but it helps enormously if they also focus on redefining their sense of identity as a calm and centred person. They can then think, "What would a calm and centred person do in this situation?" Given the huge impact stress has on our long-term health, it's imperative that we prioritise our outlook, be mindful of our self-talk and create new thoughts and beliefs about what's possible as we age.

It's rather like wanting to use the latest functionality in an Excel spreadsheet with a very out-of-date version of Microsoft Windows, or wanting to upload the latest apps to an old iPad or iPhone. We need new programming! And this is what this chapter is all about: finding easy and time-efficient ways to integrate our learning into our lives.

A belief is simply a thought we keep thinking. If we want to change our beliefs, we need to change our thoughts. By consciously choosing positive and empowering thoughts, we can reshape our beliefs, our approach to life and ultimately our sense of identity. As Louise Hay once said, "It's only a thought, and a thought can be changed."

When thinking about our later years, we want to feel optimistic, to embrace the time we have, to feel full of vitality and live life to the full. Even when we have acquired the knowledge of why and how to adopt an ageless attitude, actually implementing it takes more than the power of our good intentions.

In an episode of *The Simpsons*, the community attempts to rebuild ned Flanders' home after a hurricane destroys it. Unfortunately, their reconstruction is poorly executed, leading to the house collapsing again. In a rare display of anger, Ned confronts his neighbours, including Marge Simpson, expressing his frustration by saying: "Well, my family can't live in 'good intentions,' Marge!"

Without effective action, there are limits to our good intentions. We know we want to make some changes, but the overwhelming to-do list always takes precedence. Our best intentions can often end up on the "someday" list instead, and someday never comes.

Another reason we don't take action is that we think *"I know that."* These are the three least helpful words for ongoing development, according to one of our inspiring mentors, Paul O'Mahoney. He asks, "Do you know that, or do you do that?" and recommends getting in the habit of doing, not knowing. Knowledge is not power – applied knowledge is power.

Reading this book so far, there are probably lots of topics that you already know about. At this point, it may be worth asking, "Do

I do that?" Are there some tweaks and refinements you need to make to ensure you're living and breathing an ageless attitude?

Later in the chapter, there are lots of ideas for you to try to help you combine your life wisdom and any new insights you have learned so you can live an optimistic and vibrant life, whatever your age.

If You Do Just One Thing...

> *"Knowing is not enough, we must apply.*
> *Willing is not enough, we must do."*
>
> – Johann Wolfgang von Goethe

When life is busy, the thought of fitting something else into the day can feel overwhelming. It can take time to work out what you need to do first, and your best intentions end up on the back burner.

A great starting point we'd recommend is to focus on your self-talk. If you do just one thing, notice your thoughts and replace those that no longer serve you with more empowering ones that represent the person you want to be. Below are a few ways to do so.

The Thought Swap

Choose a recurring negative or limiting thought you've noticed. Some common ones might be:

- *"It's too late for me to change."*

- *"I'm not as sharp as I used to be."*
- *"No one really values older people anymore."*
- *"My best years are behind me."*

Ask yourself:

- *Is this thought absolutely true? 100% true?*
- *How does it make me feel or behave?*
- *What might a more empowering, compassionate version sound like?*

Here are a few examples:

- *"I've lived through enough to know that growth is always possible."*
- *"My experience and perspective are more valuable now than ever."*
- *"My best years are the ones I choose to make meaningful."*

Repeat your new thought when the old one resurfaces. In our experience, it can take a bit of repetition! It is worth it, though, and worth the effort.

Track Your Thoughts

Set a timer for three or four times throughout the day. Each time it goes off, take 30 seconds to write down what you were just thinking. Was the thought kind, helpful, curious? Or was it critical, anxious or resigned?

At the end of the day, reflect: What patterns did I notice? What would I like to shift tomorrow?

Choose a Daily Affirmation

Pick one empowering phrase to carry with you this week, like:

- *"My value is not defined by my age, but by how fully I live."*
- *"My success is measured by how much fun I'm having."*
- *"I trust my inner wisdom."*
- *"I release old stories and make space for new possibilities."*
- *"I trust the unfolding of my life."*

Write it on a Post-it or on your phone and repeat it each morning before starting your day.

Visualise the Future You

Take a few minutes to close your eyes and imagine the most vibrant, grounded, fulfilled version of yourself five years from now. Ask:

- *What does their self-talk sound like?*
- *How would they respond to challenges?*

Start practising those responses now. Your future self is simply the one you rehearse becoming.

> *"Nobody wakes up in the morning and tells you what to think about. You have the power to think whatever thoughts you like."*
>
> – Robin Banks

Every thought we think will impact our outlook, so we need to choose carefully. We also need to be mindful of our triggers. We have been committed to embracing a new outlook on ageing for a few years now, but we still find certain triggers will take us back to old disempowering thought patterns. As is often said, "Triggers are a gift, being triggered is not." Being aware of our triggers helps us to view them objectively and reduces the probability of an emotive reaction.

For example, a friend once said to Sue, "Well, the best years are behind us now." This comment touched a nerve, stirring feelings of doubt, sadness and apprehension. It triggered old thought patterns, prompting her to question whether she had made the most of her life. Had she wasted too much time? Was she being unrealistic about what was possible in the years to come? Was there even enough time left? Catching herself, Sue realised that she was placing her focus on things she couldn't control; she can't change the past and there's no way of knowing how much time she has left. She reflected, asking, "How does this thought serve me?" and "What else could I think and feel at this point to feel more hopeful about the future?" By challenging these disempowering thoughts, she began to feel a spark of clarity and optimism. She realised that her future could still be vibrant and full of possibilities, regardless of her age.

Replacing disempowering self-talk with uplifting alternatives is a cornerstone of shifting our mindset about ageing. Below are 10 common negative thoughts, along with empowering replacements, which we hope will be useful to you:

1. *"The best days are behind me."*

Empowering replacement:

"Every stage of life brings new opportunities for joy, growth and purpose."

"The best days are the ones I create for myself, starting today."

"I'm excited about my future"

Rationale: Joy and fulfilment are not bound by age; they are created through our intentions and mindset. Embrace the limitless potential of each new day to shape the life you desire.

2. *"It's all downhill from here."*

Empowering replacement:

"I have the wisdom, resilience and freedom to make this the most meaningful chapter of my life."

"I'm stronger, wiser and more capable of handling life than ever before."

"With age comes the freedom, wisdom and confidence to live more authentically than ever before."

Rationale: Ageing is not a decline; it's a journey toward greater self-awareness, freedom and purpose. Celebrate the strength and insight that come from a life well-lived. And who says "downhill" is a bad thing? If you think of it like sledging, it takes a lot of effort to trudge up the hill in the snow, but it's all worth it for that exhilarating ride down the slope!

3. "At my age, it's too late."

Empowering replacement:

"It's never too late to learn, grow or start something new."

"My age gives me the perfect perspective to tackle this with wisdom and clarity."

Rationale: Remarkable achievements can happen at any age. Let inspiring examples remind you that age is not a limitation but an advantage in making wiser, more meaningful decisions.

4. "I'm too old for that."

Empowering replacement:

"I'm exactly the right age to enjoy life fully and pursue what matters most."

"Age is just a number; enthusiasm and action keep me vibrant."

Rationale: Age is a mindset, not a barrier. Passions and joy have no expiration date. Embrace what excites and fulfils you, regardless of the number of candles on your cake.

5. "I can't keep up with younger people."

Empowering replacement:

"I bring experience and perspective that complement youthful energy."

"I'm not here to compete; I'm here to thrive on my own terms."

Rationale: The "comparison curse" can be very disempowering. Rather than comparing and contrasting, focus on collaboration. Embrace your unique strengths to complement the skillsets of younger people.

6. "My body is falling apart."

Empowering replacement:

"My body is resilient and capable; I honour it by taking care of it."

"I listen to my body and support it with kindness and care."

Rationale: Your body deserves gratitude and care for all it does. It has an amazing capacity to heal.

7. "Nobody wants to hear what I have to say."

Empowering replacement:

"My voice matters, and my experiences can inspire and guide others."

"I have a unique perspective that enriches the lives of those around me."

Rationale: Your wisdom and experience have the power to inspire, connect and leave a lasting impact. Share your perspectives with pride.

8. *"I'll never be as strong/fit/energetic as I was."*

Empowering replacement:

"Strength and energy come in many forms; I'm focused on what I can do today."

"I'm building a new kind of strength, one that comes from adaptability and persistence."

Rationale: Redefine strength and energy by focusing on progress and adaptability rather than comparisons to the past. Growth is about what you can do now.

9. *"I'm irrelevant now."*

Empowering replacement:

"My life experience is valuable, adding depth and meaning to everything I do."

"I create relevance by staying curious, engaged and open to learning."

Rationale: Relevance comes from staying active, curious and engaged in life. Your experience and openness keep you connected and meaningful in every moment.

10. "I'm fearful of getting old."

Empowering replacement:

"Ageing is a privilege that not everyone gets to experience."

"With each passing year, I have the chance to grow richer in wisdom, gratitude and love."

Rationale: Ageing is a gift that offers you the opportunity to deepen your gratitude, wisdom and connection to life's beauty. It's a journey to cherish, not to fear.

Tuning into your self-talk can be fitted into the day without it taking up too much time. Notice your self-talk when you're in a queue, waiting for a train, hanging out the washing, brushing your teeth, blow drying your hair, waiting for the kettle to boil. Some people have found that checking their self-talk every couple of hours helps them to maintain the momentum.

It's important to notice your inner dialogue with curiosity, not judgement. Be patient with yourself. A pipette of black paint in a pot of white paint isn't going to change the colour instantly. We need to be patient, knowing that in time, there will be a crucial turning point when our new thoughts and beliefs become our new default programming and old triggers no longer elicit an unwanted reaction.

Here are some ideas to try using the GRACE model from the Life Wisdom chapter. For those people who prefer to know why rather than just how, we have included studies for each letter of the framework:

GRACE as the Framework for Living the Learning

> *"Begin doing what you want to do now. We are not living in eternity. We have only this moment, sparkling like a star in our hand and melting like a snowflake."*
>
> – Francis Bacon

G - Gratitude

Cultivate gratitude for life's finite nature and the people and experiences that bring joy.

Grounding in gratitude helps shift focus to the present, fostering contentment and resilience. It helps us to focus on the positive and trains our brains to look at the possibilities.

Study: Becca Levy's research from the Ohio Longitudinal Study of Ageing and Retirement found that individuals with a positive perception of ageing lived longer than those with less favourable views.[2]

- Start or end each day by writing down three things you're grateful for. Collating a list first thing in the morning creates a great vibe for your day. Writing down what you're grateful for directly before bedtime will inform how you wake up.

- You'll notice that many will be repeated. Focus on adding something new each day. Also, think about the small or simple things you're grateful for. They are often more powerful.

- Use a gratitude jar to collect these moments and review them periodically.

- Take five minutes during a meal to mentally thank the people, nature and effort behind the food.

- On your commute, reflect on one thing that went well during the day.

R - Release

Let go of resentment, regret or burdens that no longer serve you.

Releasing past pain creates space for emotional freedom and growth.

Study: Research involving older adults assessed the impact of subliminal positive and negative messages on walking patterns, specifically the time their foot is off the ground (swing time). Positive subliminal messages led to improved physical performance, highlighting the importance of releasing negative self-talk.[3]

- Write a forgiveness letter to someone you've held a grudge against. Don't send the letter – shred or burn it to free yourself. Use visualisation techniques to imagine letting go of a burden. Remember the Deepak Chopra quote: "You don't forgive because the person deserves forgiveness, you forgive because you deserve the peace."

- Spend five minutes journaling about one limiting belief and how you can reframe it.

- Use a simple breath mantra, like "I release" on the exhale, while breathing deeply for three minutes.

A - Align

Align your actions with what truly matters most to you.

Living intentionally ensures that time and energy are invested in what supports your values and purpose.

Study: A study published in *Frontiers in Psychology* found that individuals who align their actions with personal values experience greater wellbeing and life satisfaction. Conversely, a discrepancy between one's values and actions can lead to internal conflict and reduced personal accomplishment.[4]

- Create a "values inventory," listing your top five values and how your daily actions support or contradict them.

- Start the day by identifying one action that aligns with your core values.

- Use a habit tracker to monitor how often your actions reflect what's most important to you.

C - Connection

Nurture meaningful relationships and foster compassion for others and yourself.

Love and connection are central to a fulfilling life and are often the source of our greatest joys.

Study: Research from Harvard T.H. Chan School of Public Health indicates that social connections are crucial for longevity. Socially disconnected individuals face higher risks of heart disease, stroke, anxiety, depression and dementia. Loneliness and social isolation have been shown to increase the risk of premature death by 26% and 29%, respectively.[5]

- Call or meet with a friend or family member on a frequent basis, or volunteer in your community.

- Build friendships with people from different generations.

- Make sure the people you spend the most time with also have an empowering and fun-fuelled approach to life.

- Write a heartfelt thank-you note to someone who has impacted your life.

- Practise self-compassion by speaking to yourself as you would a dear friend when you feel self-doubt.

E - Embrace

Embrace life's finite nature to live with presence, purpose and perspective.

Awareness of life's brevity can inspire us to savour each moment and make the most of our time.

Studies: An article from "Harvard Health" collated studies showing that having a sense of purpose is associated with better health outcomes, including a lower risk of heart disease and stroke. [6]

- Write down how you'd spend your time if you had only a year to live and start implementing small changes today.
- Take a five-minute walk outside and focus on the sights, sounds and sensations around you.
- Set a timer for three minutes and reflect on the question: "What matters most to me right now?"

Final Thoughts

We hope this chapter has been a useful reminder of the distinction between what we think we know and what we actually live in practice. True wisdom is lived, not just learned. At a time in history when we're fortunate to have knowledge at our fingertips, the challenge is not about learning more; it's about applying the knowledge that's most important to us so we can live life to the full. This takes focus and dedication. If you're anything like us, then you've often set out with the best of intentions, only to find yourself slipping back into familiar grooves. Knowing that yoga is a great way to keep joints flexible as we get older did not make Sue supple until she finally got into the habit of practising yoga every day!

Reaping the benefits of having a new perception of ageing is not going to spring from the pages of a book or an inspiring quote. What begins as a fleeting intention – to savour every moment, to cherish what matters, for example – only gains power with the deliberate choices we make each day, one thought and one action at a time.

There's something freeing in recognising that change isn't about grand, sweeping gestures – it's taking incremental steps to embed your learning. Regularly asking, "Do I know that, or do I do that?" can be helpful for keeping track of the knowledge you want to apply and integrate into your life. We love the Mary Oliver quote: "Tell me, what is it you plan to do with your one wild and precious life?" It helps to keep us focused on what's important and reminds us to take action!

You may like to look at how you could apply the GRACE model to help you integrate an empowering approach to living life to the full; choose a few of the "Empowering Replacements" that resonate with you, or write some of your own. It's worth the effort to keep repeating the statements until they become an integral part of your outlook and way of being.

In the next chapter, we explore how to bring a deeper sense of vitality and richness to the life you're already living, not through grand gestures, but by tuning into the sense of wonder, even in the simplest of experiences. By keeping joy, openness and curiosity alive, we can remain aware of just how precious this one life truly is.

"To know and not to do is not to know."

– Zen Proverb

CHAPTER 8
Keeping a Sense of Wonder

"Do not grow old, no matter how long you live. Never cease to stand like curious children before the great mystery into which we were born."

– Albert Einstein

In the rush of daily life, there's always something to do or somewhere to be. How often do we have the space in our lives to stop and stare up at the stars or savour a sunset? With the constant torrent of negative news headlines, is it any surprise that our sense of wonder fades away?

Our aim is to help you explore and find an empowering approach to ageing, one that honours your life wisdom, nurtures your vitality, helps you navigate the inevitable challenges and encourages you to be aligned to your true sense of meaning through your passions and living in line with your inner purpose.

You might be wondering, "What does a sense of wonder have to do with that?" Wonder often gets written off as something reserved for children or dreamers. But it's not something we outgrow; it's something we stop noticing. It doesn't disappear. It just fades into the background, hidden behind habits, responsibilities and the constant noise of everyday life.

This chapter is about bringing it back into focus. Through simple, practical ways – like moments in nature, sparks of creativity or slowing down enough to really *see* what's around you – you'll begin to reconnect with a part of yourself that's always been there. A sense of wonder isn't just a luxury; it connects us to feeling more present, more uplifted and more alive in every stage of life.

This chapter invites you to reclaim the childlike qualities that allow life to feel expansive, exciting and filled with possibility, without losing the depth of wisdom and perspective that comes with age.

Many of us have been conditioned to believe that ageing means becoming more serious, more realistic, more worldly and as a result, we can feel a little jaded. Wonder, playfulness and curiosity are often dismissed as qualities reserved for the young. But what if the key to feeling ageless isn't in resisting time, but in rekindling our ability to see the world with fresh eyes?

Deepak Chopra puts it beautifully: "Be childlike, not childish. To be childlike is to be innocent, curious and full of wonder." Being childlike means embracing curiosity, awe and playfulness, qualities that keep life vibrant and meaningful at any age. It is about looking at the sky and marvelling at the changing colours of dusk, getting lost in a piece of music that stirs something deep inside or feeling a sense of magic in the everyday moments we often overlook.

Tapping into a sense of wonder is not about pretending to be young; it is about choosing to stay alive to life's magic. It is about remaining open, engaged and enchanted by the beauty that surrounds us. In the pages ahead, we'll explore how to awaken this sense of wonder, not just in the abstract, but through your senses, your daily experiences and your approach to life itself. You'll discover that wonder is not something lost with age, but something that, when nurtured, deepens and becomes even more meaningful with age.

Acting Our Age

When your mind is full of your ever-growing list of commitments, family worries and looming work deadlines, there's little headspace left for seeing the world with a sense of awe. Also, without often realising it, we can deny ourselves a sense of child-like wonder because we believe, for some reason, that we should "act our age." Here are a few comments we heard in conversation recently when we were asking friends their thoughts on having a sense of wonder:

> "Wonder is for children, not adults."
>
> "Life is too busy – there's no time to focus on wonder."
>
> "It's all a bit Pollyanna to me."
>
> "At my age, I already know what life is about. There's not much left to be amazed by."

Yet when we let go of that constrictive programming, we allow spontaneity and fun to flow. We get back in touch with our inner sense of ageless joy.

One of our favourite films is *Enchanted April*. At the beginning of the film, Joan Plowright's character, Mrs. Fisher, clings to the rigid proprieties of age, her every word and posture a quiet insistence that she must remain as she has always been: dignified, composed, untouchable by whimsy. When confronted with the idea of joy, of spontaneity, her response is firm: "I won't have it." Yet, as the Italian spring unfolds around her and she starts to feel more relaxed in the company of the others, she lets go of her ingrained principles.

One day, almost without thinking, she reaches for a set of watercolours. At first, her hand hesitates. It is foolish, indulgent, not something a woman of her age and standing should do. But then, she gives herself permission to find some paper and a brush. Opening up the tin again, she starts to paint a geranium on the page. In that moment, she is no longer Mrs. Fisher, guardian of the past; she is a child again, wide-eyed, smiling with contentment and discovering the world anew.

The Science of Awe:
A Boost for Wellbeing and Connection

One of the most powerful elements of wonder is awe, that deep, expansive feeling we experience when we witness something vast, beautiful or profoundly moving. A growing body of neuroscience research shows that awe triggers the release of dopamine and oxytocin, two key neurochemicals that enhance wellbeing and strengthen social bonds.

In one study, older adults were encouraged to seek out experiences of wonder – in nature, architecture and art – during their daily walks. After an eight-week period, those who intentionally cultivated awe reported greater feelings of joy, gratitude and connection, along with reduced anxiety and stronger emotional resilience, which is a key marker of healthy ageing.[1]

Another study found that awe was the most powerful of the positive emotions for reducing inflammation markers linked to chronic diseases such as arthritis and heart disease.[2] Less inflammation, of course, means better health over time.

So, the effects of awe go beyond momentary pleasure. It creates lasting changes in how we perceive ourselves and the world, making us feel more connected, present and engaged in life. Whether it's staring at a star-filled sky, listening to a breathtaking piece of music or witnessing an act of kindness, awe has the power to reset our perspective and bring us back to a place of wonder.

The Hawkins Scale of Consciousness, developed by psychiatrist Dr. David R. Hawkins, maps human emotions and states of awareness on a logarithmic scale from 0 to 1,000, where each level corresponds to a specific energy frequency.[3] At the lower end, below 200, lie emotions like shame (20), fear (100) and anger (150), which Hawkins argued drain energy and limit perception, as measured through applied kinesiology and corroborated by studies on psychophysiology.

Above 200, the scale shifts to positive states like courage (200), love (500) and enlightenment (700+), with frequencies that uplift and expand awareness. Awe, which Hawkins placed around 450-500 alongside joy and peace, resonates at a high vibrational level, aligning with research showing that awe-inducing experiences – like marvelling at nature or art – reduce stress hormones, boost oxytocin and activate the prefrontal cortex, enhancing creativity and connection. By cultivating awe, we tap into this higher energy bandwidth, not just feeling good but fundamentally shifting how we engage with the world, as Hawkins' framework suggests our consciousness shapes our reality.

What You See Is What You Become

In our modern world, where distressing news cycles run 24/7, we are subtly trained to focus on what is alarming rather than what is wonderful. In Chapter 2, we explored the mind-body connection. Dr. Christiane Northrup encapsulated the impact of this succinctly when she said, "Over time, the images, thoughts and emotions we experience are programming our biology." Many of us have absorbed the belief that if we do not pay attention to every crisis, every catastrophe, we are being irresponsible. In reality, a steady diet of fear and despair rewires our nervous system, floods us with stress hormones and dulls our ability to see joy. We can become world-weary. A few seconds of appreciating a sunset cannot undo the effects of hours spent bombarded by the distressing news reports.

Where we place our focus determines how we feel, how we age and how we experience the world. By consciously choosing to delight in the simple pleasures of life and immerse ourselves in moments of curiosity, beauty and gratitude, we rewire our minds and bodies for joy.

Don't take our word for it! We found that when we first came across this concept, it sounded plausible in theory, but what about in practice? It's one of those concepts that you'll only ever truly appreciate when you've applied it. We could not have imagined how powerful this is, so we would highly recommend that you give it a try. You'll be amazed at how differently you'll feel.

In the last few months, we have got into the habit of asking ourselves, "*What's wonderful about this moment?*" Our goal was to be more mindful of our thoughts and to keep a sense of perspective. On tough days when nothing seemed to be going to plan, asking what was wonderful about the moment initially wound us up and our inner dialogue did not give the politest of responses!

Over time, the question helped us to take a step back and look at what we could learn from the moment, however unwanted the situation. Just asking the question in those rotten moments simply made us laugh. Like Captain Pyke in *Star Trek: Strange New Worlds* said to Spock, "Sometimes the situation is so bad you just have to laugh." This new habit has proved useful in looking at the upsides of a situation, even in moments we might once have seen only in a negative light. It's amazing how resourceful our minds can be in finding the positives and valuable insights.

If you want to give this a try, be patient with yourself. You may find yourself irritated or cynical when asking, "What's wonderful about this moment?" We felt exactly the same at first. When you're tired, frustrated or overwhelmed, the last thing your mind wants is a forced silver lining. So, when you're having a tough day and nothing's going as you would like, you may prefer to pause and ask, "What's still okay?" Don't pressure yourself to find something profound or perfect. Just look for one small thing that's not terrible – it could be sipping a decent cup of tea, the train is on time, someone holding the door open for you with a smile or simply acknowledging the fact that you're keeping going, even on a tough day. Start there. The goal isn't to deny your feelings; it's to gradually shift your focus so your mind begins to notice the good that's also present.

Triggering a Sense of Wonder

As we write this chapter in the final week of February 2025, there's a rare alignment of the seven planets – Mercury, Venus, Mars, Jupiter, Saturn, Uranus and Neptune – that won't be seen again until 2040. This alignment serves as a poignant reminder to pause, look up from our daily routines and marvel at the cosmos above. Such moments not only provide perspective on our place in the universe but also underscore the transient nature of these events, urging us to cherish and capture them.

This month also marks the 35th anniversary of the iconic "Pale Blue Dot" photograph. As Voyager 1 drifted toward the edges of our solar system, its power waning after more than a decade in space, NASA scientists debated how to make the most of its remaining energy. There were still scientific measurements to take, data to collect, but Carl Sagan had another idea. He urged them to turn the spacecraft around, just once, for one final photograph. It was an unusual request. Voyager was nearly 4 billion miles from home, its mission nearly complete. But NASA agreed, and on February 14, 1990, as the spacecraft prepared to leave our planetary neighbourhood forever, it snapped a single, extraordinary image. Against the vast blackness of space, Earth appeared as nothing more than a pale blue dot, a tiny, fragile speck suspended in a sunbeam.

That image changed the way we see ourselves. It was humbling, a reminder of how small we are in the grand expanse of the universe. But it was also profound. From that tiny dot had come love, art, discovery, science, philosophy, every human experience, every act of courage and kindness. In that moment, Voyager 1, an ageing spacecraft with dwindling power, gave us a gift of immeasurable wonder.

Isn't that, in some ways, the essence of ageing well? Like Voyager, some of us may feel we are running low on energy, past the prime of our mission, wondering how best to spend the time we have left. Perhaps the most powerful thing we can do is what Sagan proposed: to turn around, to look at life with fresh eyes, to capture something beautiful, to remind ourselves there is still time to create, to marvel, to inspire. The Pale Blue Dot reminds us that wonder is not just for the young; it is for anyone willing to turn back and see life with fresh eyes.

Much like Voyager's last glance homeward, the current planetary alignment encourages us to seize fleeting opportunities to reflect, appreciate and find wonder in the universe. These experiences enrich our lives, fostering a sense of connection and timeless curiosity.

When Stu was a teenager, he was captivated by Carl Sagan's TV series *Cosmos*. It catalysed a lifelong passion for astronomy. Carl Sagan had a rare gift for making even the most complex concepts feel accessible and fascinating. He never spoke down to his audience; instead, he invited them to join him in curiosity, as if unlocking the mysteries of the cosmos together.

His evident love of his subject, storytelling brilliance and ability to frame science as an ongoing adventure made people feel not just informed, but uplifted, as though they, too, were part of something grand and meaningful. He didn't just teach facts, he sparked wonder and reminded us that questioning, exploring and marvelling are lifelong pursuits. His inspiring approach to life is encapsulated in this quote: "Somewhere, something incredible is waiting to be known." A few years ago, we watched the series again. As well as being awe-inspiring, it was a bit of a wake-up call for Stu as he realised how much his teenage sense of wonder had faded over the years. It was then that he made a pact with himself to reignite it. Making that decision has been great for his outlook on life. It's also impacted others, and his infectious enthusiasm has often prompted friends to say how envious they are of him and how it's inspired them to look at life differently.

The Never-Ending Unfolding of Wonder

In his book *Zen Mind, Beginner's Mind*, Shunryu Suzuki emphasises the value of approaching life with openness, eagerness and a lack of preconceptions. He famously said, "In the beginner's mind, there are many possibilities, but in the expert's mind, there are few." This mindset frees us from the trap of thinking we've arrived at some ultimate understanding, urging us instead to remain perpetual students of life.

This idea truly resonates with us. In our own experience, the people who seem the oldest, regardless of age, are often the ones who've become fixed in their thinking. There's a rigidity to their worldview, a sense that they've stopped being curious or willing to see things differently. On the other hand, those who come across as youthful, vibrant and full of life tend to remain open. They ask questions, they listen, they adapt and they show a genuine interest in the new. We've come to believe that staying young isn't just about how we move or look, it's about how open we are to developing further, to shifting our perspective and to recognising that there's always more to learn. This is the essence of "beginner's mind," not naivety, but humility, curiosity and a willingness to meet each moment with fresh perspectives.

Suzuki's insight dovetails beautifully with the recognition that at the heart of maintaining a sense of wonder is the realisation that we will never reach the end of discovery – about the world, about ourselves or about life itself. Every question answered opens another door, every new insight invites further exploration. While Stu was inspired by Carl Sagan and *Cosmos* in the early 80s, Sue was transfixed by the TV series, *The Ascent of Man*, presented by the incredible polymath Jacob Bronowski. His thoughtful, articulate and profoundly engaging style was captivating. Similar to Carl Sagan, he had a rare capacity to make complex ideas accessible without dumbing them down. The way he traced humanity's journey through science, art and ideas sparked Sue's lifelong thirst for learning. A quote from the series goes, "There is no absolute knowledge. And those who claim it, whether they are scientists or dogmatists, open the door to tragedy. All information is imperfect. We have to treat it with humility." This humility, the understanding that there is always another layer to uncover, is liberating and empowering. Together with the beginner's mindset, we can be endlessly curious. This prevents us from becoming closed-minded and stagnating. It frees us to live with an ageless attitude.

When you think about how children approach the world, they don't assume they already know everything. They ask why, again and again, because they understand that knowledge is limitless. Somewhere along the way, many of us stop asking, believing we've already figured out what life is about. But what if we rekindled that childlike mindset? What if we embraced, as Bronowski suggests, the idea that there is no final truth, only a continuous unfolding of new possibilities?

Wonder flourishes when we let go of the need for certainty and instead embrace the joy of discovery; whether it's learning something new, experiencing an unexpected moment of beauty or simply shifting our perspective to see the extraordinary in the ordinary. By choosing to stay curious, open and humble, we keep our minds alive and engaged. We make space for awe, for learning and for the deep appreciation that life is not something to be solved but something to be experienced with endless fascination.

After Sue's dad died, there was the inevitable numbness of trying to make sense of the world without your loved one in it. In previous years, walking in the woods and seeing the bluebells would have filled her with joy, but not that year. She found herself looking down at the ground, lost in her thoughts, oblivious to the iridescent blue. Upset that her dad would never walk through the woods again, she started to question what life is all about. She thought of all the countries that her dad had wanted to visit and the ambitions he didn't get the chance to achieve. She was feeling guilty that she was still in a position to aspire towards a life that her parents had not had the opportunity to live, to see amazing places in the world and to learn new things. Without realising it at the time, she avoided setting aspirational goals. Even when she realised that she was imprisoning herself in her comfort zone, she seemed to find plenty of excuses as to why she hadn't set any meaningful goals. Then one evening, watching the film *Shirley Valentine* starring Pauline Collins, she suddenly woke up:

"I've led such a little life. And even that will be over pretty soon. I have... allowed myself to lead this little life when inside me there was so much more. And it's all gone unused. And now it never will be. Why do we get all this life if we don't ever use it?"

Hearing these words reminded Sue that she needed to dare to pursue her dreams and embrace the years ahead with wonder again. Even though there was still a part of her that felt extremely sad that her parents were no longer in a position to realise their dreams, she realised that this was not a legitimate reason not to set challenging goals. Her parents' optimism, openness to new ideas, sense of fun and amazing capacity to see the magic in the simplest of things reminded her that they would much prefer their children to live a full life rather than a little one full of regret. It was at that moment that Sue gave herself permission to dream again, to expand her life goals and ambitions, one of which was to write this book.

Finding Magic in the Everyday

One winter's evening, about 12 years ago, Sue had popped in to see her parents. Her dad had created a blazing fire in the back garden, and her mum had made the most luxurious hot chocolate. Sitting with blankets over their knees, they sipped their drinks without the need to speak that often, lost in their thoughts and mesmerised by the flickering flames. For some reason, sitting by the fire that evening, Sue thought about the fleeting nature of life. Robert Brault's words came to her mind: *"Enjoy the little things, for one day you may look back and realise they were the big things."* Looking back now, she has no idea what it was about that particular evening that made her want to capture it and absorb the magic of sharing this simple pleasure of being together. The following autumn, Sue's dad was diagnosed with small-cell lung cancer and died just a few months later. Whenever she misses her parents, she thinks back to that magical evening of simply being in their company.

She is acutely aware of how many of Robert Brault's "little things" have escaped her notice when she's been busy getting on with life. One of our fabulous mentors, Paul O'Mahoney, encapsulated this perfectly recently when he said, "Life is so incredible, yet in our minds we're constantly playing chess with ourselves." We get lost in planning our next move, rather than acknowledging how privileged we are to be alive.

William Morris said, "The secret to happiness lies in taking a genuine interest in daily life." While we often associate wonder with grand, awe-inspiring moments, true wonder is just as present in the simplest of experiences: the scent of the garden after rainfall, the way frost glistens in the sunlight, the crisp, clean feeling of freshly laundered sheets. As Marcel Proust once said, "The real voyage of discovery consists not in seeking new landscapes, but in having new eyes."

We often feel we need to travel the world to amazing places like the Niagara Falls or the Great Wall of China to experience a sense of wonder. However, we can do it closer to home as well by becoming deeply present, pausing so we can truly see, hear and feel the world around us.

Here are some of our ideas:

Be a tourist in your own town. Take a walking tour, visit a museum or gallery you've never explored or stop to read the plaques and signs you usually walk past. Try seeing your town through the eyes of someone who's never been there before.

Practise a wonder walk. Go on a slow walk, perhaps taking a different route. Set yourself a goal to notice five things you've never noticed before. Look up at rooftops, down at patterns in the pavement or at how sunlight shines through the trees. Take photos of what catches your eye.

Watch the sky. Spend a few minutes watching clouds float by. Take the time to look up at the stars. Notice all the changing colours of a sunset, knowing that no other sunset will be the same.

Visit a local park. Even a small green space can feel magical when you approach it with childlike curiosity. Sit quietly, noticing the leaves sway in the breeze, tune into the sound of children playing, dogs barking, the squeak of the swings. Notice smells, textures and colours around you.

Attend a local event you'd usually skip. It could be a craft fair, a lecture at the library or a local concert. Immersing yourself in something new can reignite interests and connect with new people in your community.

Mindful mornings. Start your day by opening a window and listening. Notice birdsong, bees buzzing, the wind in the trees, the way the light falls on a particular spot and the shapes of shadows.

Walking a dog. When you're out with your dog or you're watching dogs out on a walk, watch the way they are completely in the moment, sniffing, jumping in and out of puddles and treating everyone they meet as a new playmate. Their sense of wonder is contagious.

Embrace the art of flânerie. Wander your local streets with no destination in mind. Sit in a café and watch the world go by. This French concept celebrates the joy of observing, meandering and noticing beauty in the ordinary bustle of everyday life.

The ordinary becomes extraordinary when we give it our attention. A child's fascination with a puddle, the intricate veins of a fallen leaf, the rhythm of waves rolling onto the shore. These are reminders that wonder does not have to be a rare luxury but is instead intricately woven into the fabric of everyday life.

The Wonder Spectrum

When you're going through a particularly challenging chapter of your life, focusing on a sense of wonder is likely to be unthinkable and unattainable. At such times, it's useful to focus on taking incremental steps towards where you want to be, so you don't feel stuck and you know you're moving in the right direction. We hope the spectrum below will help you get in touch with how you're feeling in a given moment. We've also included tips on how to move up the scale a few steps at a time.

From Disenchantment to Wonder

0 - Complete disenchantment. You feel utterly detached from life's magic. The world seems predictable, dull or exhausting. You might think, "I've seen it all," or "What's the point?" Beauty, novelty and possibility feel out of reach, and even small joys are overshadowed by apathy or fatigue.

2 - Deep world-weariness. You're stuck in a rut, sceptical of change or surprises. Life feels like a repetitive chore. You might notice yourself dismissing new experiences with thoughts like, "It won't be worth it," or "I'm too old for that."

4 - Mild cynicism. You're functioning but uninspired. Things that once sparked curiosity, like nature, people or ideas, now feel ordinary. You might catch yourself saying, "That's just how it is," or brushing off excitement as naivety.

6 - Neutral curiosity. You're open but not amazed. You might notice something interesting, a sunset, a conversation, but it doesn't linger or lift you. You're coasting, neither weary nor wondrous, perhaps briefly thinking, "That's nice," but then quickly moving onto another thought.

8 - Growing wonder. You're rediscovering life's spark. You feel a pull toward exploration: trying a new hobby, asking questions or pausing to marvel at small things. Thoughts like, "I wonder how that works," or "That's pretty amazing," bubble up naturally.

10 - Full childlike wonder. You're alive with awe and possibility. The world feels fresh, vibrant and full of mystery, no matter your age. You might laugh at a quirky detail, stare at the stars or feel fired up about learning something new, thinking, "Wow, isn't this incredible?"

Depending on what's going on in our lives, we've all probably experienced every scale on this spectrum. Our goal is to move you closer to 10 as frequently as possible. When we're keen to feel a sense of awe again, we can get impatient with ourselves. If you're anything like us, you probably think, "I should have mastered this by now." It doesn't matter where you are on the scale; the important thing is nudging up the scale in manageable steps. Here are a few tips for helping you move up a few notches at a time:

From Complete Disenchantment (0) to Deep World-Weariness (2)

At 0, life feels like a slog – everything's dulled out. The goal here is just to crack the door open to possibility, even a tiny bit.

Start with one sense: Pick something simple like the smell of coffee, the sound of rain or the feel of a soft blanket. Focus on it for 30 seconds without judgment. It's not about forcing wonder; it's about allowing it to be more evident.

Vent it out: Write or say aloud one thing that's weighing you down – "I'm sick of this routine" – then let it sit. Sometimes naming the heaviness makes it less suffocating, inching you toward 2.

Tiny defiance: Do one small thing that breaks the "What's the point?" script or the feeling of apathy. It might be stepping outside for a minute or flipping on a song you used to love.

From Deep World-Weariness (2) to Mild Cynicism (4)

At 2, you're stuck in a loop of "same old, same old" or just feeling a bit jaded. The aim is to loosen that scepticism just enough to see a flicker of potential.

Challenge the rut: Pick one routine thing, like your commute or a meal, and tweak it slightly. Take a different route, add a random spice. It's not about fireworks; it's about disrupting the "nothing changes" vibe.

Borrow someone else's eyes: Watch a child, a pet or even a stranger react to something, a bug, a cloud or a laugh. Their perspective might nudge you to think differently.

Recall a past spark: Think of a time you felt even slightly curious, years ago, maybe. Don't overanalyse it; just let the memory sit there. It's a reminder that 4 isn't impossible.

From Mild Cynicism (4) to Neutral Curiosity (6)

At 4, you're coasting but uninspired. Nothing's bad, but nothing's exciting. The trick is to coax out a bit of active interest.

Ask a dumb question: Look at something ordinary, a tree or a gadget and wonder something silly like, "Why's it shaped like that?" or "Who thought to invent that?" No need to answer; just let the question take your thinking in a new direction.

Try a micro-adventure: Spend 5 minutes exploring. Peek down a side street, Google a random fact, flip to a book page you've never read. It doesn't take a lot of effort, but this can take your outlook or thoughts in a new direction.

Spot one good thing: Before the day ends, name one thing that wasn't terrible: a decent sandwich, a funny line you overheard. It's a gentle push past "That's just how it is."

From Neutral Curiosity (6) to Growing Wonder (8)

At 6, you're open but not gripped by awe. Here, you're building momentum toward real engagement.

Chase the wow factor: Next time something catches your eye, like an unusual bird or a rare cloud formation, don't let it drop. Look it up, watch it longer, tell someone about it. Turn "That's interesting" into "I want to know more."

Make it hands-on: Try something small but active. For example, sketch a flower, cook a new recipe, fix something. Doing wakes up wonder better than just watching.

Pause the rush: When you notice something inspiring like a sunset or a moving piece of music, acknowledge it either inwardly by noticing your thoughts or actually saying out loud, "Wow, I'm glad I took the time to acknowledge that."

From Growing Wonder (8) to Full Childlike Wonder (10)

From 8 to 10, it's about amplifying that spark into unrestrained awe. These work from lower levels too, if you're feeling bold!

Play like a child: Do something just for the fun of it. Jump in a puddle, kick through the fallen autumn leaves, build a tiny tower of rocks, chase a butterfly.

Hunt the mystery: Pick something you don't get, for example, stars and planets, the dance of bees, how engines work and dive in like it's a treasure hunt. Let "I wonder" turn into "Wow, that's incredible!"

Share the wow: When something hits you like a view or a story, tell someone with all the enthusiasm you've got. Their reaction, or just the act of sharing, can catapult you to 10.

As mentioned above, these steps are like a ladder – small rungs, not giant leaps. Someone at 0 doesn't need to aim for 10 right away; even 2 is progress. It's all about meeting yourself where you currently are and gently nudging the dial up.

Tapping Into Wonder Through the Senses

> *"The world is full of magic things, patiently waiting for our senses to grow sharper."*
>
> – W.B. Yeats

Using all our senses can be a great way to tap into our sense of wonder. Each of us favours particular senses. Have you noticed what usually triggers your sense of awe? For example, are you more visual than auditory? Do you tend to be captivated by a painting or sunset far more than being moved by a piece of music? Tune into what sparks your sense and wonder. We hope the suggestions below will help you to, as Yeats suggests, sharpen those senses that are not used so frequently.

Sight: Seeing the world with fresh eyes.

Pause and observe: Take a moment each day to stop and truly look at something: sunlight filtering through leaves, the intricate pattern of a flower, the twinkle of city lights.

Use "beginner's eyes": Pretend you're seeing something for the first time. Imagine describing it to someone who has never seen it before.

Seek beauty in the ordinary: Notice the play of shadows on the wall, the way raindrops run down a window or the vibrant colours of fruit at a market.

Sunsets and stargazing: Watching the sky change colours at dusk or lying under a blanket of stars can instantly awaken a sense of awe.

Sound: The magic of music and silence.

Listen to music that moves you: Some songs or pieces of music can stop you in your tracks – classical symphonies, jazz improvisations, ancient chants or even the sounds of nature. Let yourself feel the music, not just hear it.

Tune into natural sounds: Close your eyes and focus on birdsong, the rustling of leaves, the waves crashing on the shore or the patter of rain on the roof.

Try deep listening: Instead of just hearing background noise, fully immerse yourself in a sound. Try listening to a piece of music with no distractions and notice every instrument, every shift in melody or change of key.

Enjoy silence: Sometimes, wonder comes from the contrast between sound and silence. Find a quiet place and simply be.

Touch: Feeling the world around you.

Focus on textures: Run your fingers over different surfaces – tree bark, smooth pebbles, the softness of a pet's fur, the coolness of water.

Be present in simple actions: Feel the warmth of the sun on your skin, the sensation of walking barefoot on grass or sand, the contrast of hot and cold when sipping a drink.

Get creative: Engaging in activities like painting, pottery, knitting or gardening connects you to the tactile world in a deeply satisfying way.

Hug more: Physical touch, whether hugging a loved one, a pet or even wrapping yourself in a cosy blanket, can evoke deep feelings of connection and warmth.

Taste: Savouring the world.

Eat mindfully: Instead of rushing through meals, take time to truly taste each bite. Notice the flavours, textures and aromas.

Try a new flavour: Choose something on the menu you have never ordered before. Try a new cuisine or a new ingredient. Sometimes, just savouring your favourite meal can be an instant way to experience wonder.

Savour something simple: A perfectly ripe peach, a piece of dark chocolate melting on your tongue or a sip of rich coffee can be a moment of pure delight.

Cook with curiosity: Experimenting with spices, herbs and ingredients you've never used before or trying a new recipe can awaken a playful sense of wonder in the kitchen.

The six tastes: Try to eat all of the six tastes every day and notice each of them: sweet, sour, salty, bitter, astringent and pungent.

Smell: Scents that evoke memories and magic.

Reconnect with nature's fragrance: The scent of jasmine on a summer evening, pine trees in a forest or the salty breeze of the sea can instantly shift your mood.

Use aromatherapy: Essential oils like lavender, citrus or sandalwood can transport you to different emotional states. Find the oils you have an affinity with and use them in diffusers or in the bath.

Notice everyday scents: Freshly brewed coffee, baking bread, the pages of an old book – savour the small, familiar smells that bring comfort and nostalgia.

Breathe it in deeply: When you encounter a scent that stirs something in you, take a moment to close your eyes and inhale deeply, letting it fully register.

Bringing it All Together: A Multi-Sensory Experience

Go on a wonder walk: Take a slow walk and engage all five senses. Notice colours, listen to sounds, touch different textures, breathe in the scents and if possible, taste something fresh like a piece of fruit.

Create a "wonder ritual": Light a candle with a beautiful scent, play inspiring music, hold a warm cup of tea in your hands and savour the moment with full presence.

Keep a "sense of wonder" journal: Write down at least one sensory experience each day that made you pause and feel amazed.

If some of these suggestions feel out of reach, unfamiliar or even a little indulgent, that's completely understandable. We felt the same way to begin with. You may find yourself thinking, *"I don't have time for this,"* or *"It sounds lovely, but I just don't feel that way."* Many of us have spent years in "doing" mode, rushing through days without pausing to really *feel* them. It's a bit like being on a train journey. You're travelling through incredible landscapes, but you're glued to your phone, immersed in a book or tapping away on your laptop. You don't notice the wildflowers by the tracks, the shifting light or the people around you. Hours pass, and you reach your destination, but you didn't really experience the journey.

The busyness of life can mean that we move through our days on autopilot, missing the beauty, the wonder and the quiet miracles happening all around us. Reconnecting with your senses is like looking out of the window on the train and really seeing the view. The journey doesn't change, but your experience of it does. Reconnecting with wonder can feel awkward at first, especially if you're out of the habit of slowing down. Start gently. Choose just one sense to focus on each day, or even each week. Let your curiosity guide you. You don't have to force a sense of awe. Over time, you'll find that the more you notice, the more there is to notice. And the smallest moments, the scent of rain, the feel of sunlight on your skin, might start to take on a quiet kind of magic of their own.

Final Thoughts

> *"We don't stop playing because we grow old; we grow old because we stop playing."*
>
> – George Bernard Shaw

The demands, time constraints and stresses of daily life, accompanied by the continual joy vacuum of the news headlines, can lead to feeling world-weary as the norm. Viewing the world with a sense of wonder can feel unrealistic. However, as you've seen, far from being an indulgence, wonder is a biological necessity. It keeps the mind open, the heart engaged and enables the body to thrive. Science confirms what many of us instinctively know. Curiosity, awe and playfulness don't fade with age; they help us stay truly alive.

Life is full of contrasts with inevitable ups and downs. Challenging chapters constrain our capacity to tap into our sense of wonder. It's often those setbacks that take us in a new direction and lead us to an even better outcome that we otherwise would not have known. For us, it was often only in hindsight that we could see how a tough time in our lives led either to a much better outcome or was a valuable lesson to learn. Asking "What's wonderful about this moment?" when life isn't going to plan or we're feeling stressed, has helped us to pause and to be an objective observer. Looking at the situation from a new perspective has enabled us to be more resourceful with the solutions we devise.

Given that we only have a finite number of days on the planet, it's important to reflect on how much of our time we are assigning to seeing the wonder in things and how much time we're sleepwalking through life. Focusing on wonder is a choice. By making small shifts, staying curious, seeking out moments of awe and embracing a playful spirit, we can cultivate a sense of wonder that enhances not just our mood but our overall health and longevity. Starting this chapter with an Einstein quote, it only feels right to finish with his wise philosophy on life: *"There are only two ways to live your life. One is as though nothing is a miracle. The other is as though everything is a miracle."*

Conclusion: Ageing as a Journey of Empowerment

"The only way to make sense out of change is to plunge into it, move with it and join the dance."

– Alan Watts

As we come to the end of this book, we hope you feel a shift – a spark of possibility that wasn't there when you first turned these pages. Perhaps you began this journey with a quiet unease about ageing, something to put up with and out of your control. Or maybe you intuitively questioned the fear-based paradigm that being older inevitably means a decline in health and losing your spark, so you were looking for evidence to validate your perception. Alternatively, you may have thought that the way you age hinged solely on diet, supplements, fitness regimes or the luck of genetics.

Our aim has been to show you that ageing is so much more than that and, crucially, that it's far more within your control than you might have imagined. And perhaps most importantly, you've discovered that ageing is not something that just happens to you, it's something you can shape with awareness and intention.

Ideally, we'd love for this to be far more than a spark or small shift in your approach to your later years and that the old paradigm of ageing you were reminded of in Chapter 1 now feels completely alien to you!

We live in a time when the global population is ageing at an unprecedented rate. We're also seeing a growing awareness of mental and emotional wellbeing, and a collective desire to live not just longer, but better. This is a moment of amazing opportunity: a chance to redefine what it means to grow older, to move beyond the outdated stereotypes of decline and irrelevance and to create a new story of vitality, purpose and joy.

By embracing the ideas in this book, you're not just shaping your own future; you're contributing to a cultural shift that will benefit your family and friends, and the generations to come. Imagine a world where ageing is celebrated as a time of wisdom, creativity and contribution, rather than feared as a time of loss.

We also want to acknowledge that this journey isn't always easy. Ageing, like life itself, comes with challenges, some expected, some unforeseen. But what we've learned, through our own painful experiences and through the wisdom we've gained, is that challenges don't define us; how we respond to them does. By choosing to approach ageing with optimism, by harnessing the power of your thoughts and emotions and by living with purpose, passion and wonder, you can navigate any challenge with grace and emerge stronger, wiser and more fully yourself.

Briefly, to recap:

In Chapter 1, Perception of Ageing, we examined how society, media and cultural conditioning have shaped our views of growing older, often casting it as something to fear or fight. We challenged that outdated paradigm to see ageing as a journey of growth and opportunity rather than loss.

In Chapter 2, Mind Body Connection, we explored the extraordinary power of your thoughts and emotions to influence your biochemistry, revealing how your mindset can literally change your body's ageing process.

Chapter 3, Life Wisdom, encouraged you to tap into the incredible reservoir of wisdom and experience you've accumulated over the years, treating it as a source of strength and vitality.

Chapter 4, Know Thyself, invited you to tune into your unique needs and embrace your authentic self, guided by David Bowie's wisdom that ageing is a process of becoming who you were always meant to be. We also covered the concept of bio-individuality, emphasising that there's no one-size-fits-all approach to ageing well – only the path that's right for you.

Chapter 5, Navigating Life's Challenges, provided ideas and practical ways to face some of the typical trials of later life, such as bereavement, caring for elderly parents or managing health issues with resourcefulness and resilience.

In Chapter 6, Purpose and Passion, we explored the importance of aligning with what lights you up from within – the unique contribution only you can offer. We also looked at how following your passions keeps you energised, connected and joyfully engaged in life.

Chapter 7, Nothing Is Learned Until It Is Lived, focused on how true transformation does not come from knowledge alone but from living it. It offered practical tips on how you can apply your learning so that living with an ageless attitude becomes an integral part of your life.

And finally, in Chapter 8, Keeping a Sense of Wonder, we delved into how rekindling childlike curiosity and awe can help you stay vibrant, present and deeply engaged with life. No matter your age, approaching each day with openness and a sense of discovery can infuse your later years with renewed meaning and joy.

What ties all of this together is that, in our view, mastering the art of ageing isn't about resisting change or clinging to youth; it's about embracing the fullness of who you are at this point of your life, supported by the insights you have gained and having a range of resources and practices to help you live your best life. There is no single path, no one-size-fits-all formula.

How you age is influenced by how you live, how you think, how you connect and how you choose to show up for yourself each day. It's a story you co-author with every thought you choose, every emotion you nurture and every moment you embrace with intention. As you'll have seen from our experience, this isn't a linear step-by-step process. Instead, it's a dynamic, evolving journey. It unfolds through daily choices, small shifts in perspective, the meaning you create along the way and the courage to keep returning to yourself with compassion and curiosity.

In closing, thank you for taking the time to read this book. We truly hope that you've gained some useful perspectives and practical ideas to implement. At the very least, we hope you now know your later years don't need to be left to chance. They can be a vibrant, purposeful and deeply fulfilling chapter – one you have the power to define.

You'll find a selection of some of our favourite tools and inspirations in the Further Resources chapter, along with a free, online Companion Guide designed to support and inspire you.

We wish you every success in defining your later years and living every day you have on the planet to the full. As C.S. Lewis once said, "You are never too old to set another goal or to dream a new dream."

We hope this book has triggered some new thoughts and ideas on how you'd like to define and live your life, to embrace the future, to set some new goals and dream new dreams.

Further Resources

Companion Guide

To help you put the ideas in this book into practice, we've created a free Companion Guide filled with reflection prompts, space to journal, exercises from each chapter and resources we couldn't fit into the book.

You'll find the Companion Guide and far more resources on our website www.getstrongfitandhappy.com. You can also email us at info@getstrongfitandhappy.com with "Ageless Attitude Companion Guide" in the subject line. We'd love to welcome you into our growing community of like-minded souls embracing ageing with purpose, vitality and joy.

Here are some brilliant resources that we hope will prove valuable to you:

Robin Banks – Mind Power and Personal Mastery

Robin Banks is an international speaker and mindset coach best known for teaching the Mind Power method developed by John

Kehoe. His work focuses on the power of thoughts and beliefs to shape reality, with a vibrant, motivating style. Ideal if you want to explore how to intentionally direct your thinking and rewire limiting patterns.

Website: https://robinbanksmindpower.com

Dr. Joe Dispenza – Neuroscience, Meditation & Transformation

Dr. Joe Dispenza combines cutting-edge neuroscience with ancient wisdom to teach people how to rewire their brains, change their beliefs and create a new personal reality. His work is especially useful for those interested in using meditation and intention to improve health, break old habits and embrace personal evolution.

Website: https://drjoedispenza.com

Brad Yates – EFT/Tapping for Emotional and Mental Wellbeing

Known as "Tap with Brad," Brad Yates is a popular Emotional Freedom Techniques (EFT) practitioner who helps people reduce stress, release limiting beliefs and shift their mindset using the power of tapping. His YouTube channel features hundreds of guided videos and is a valuable tool for emotional resilience and self-healing.

Website: https://www.tapwithbrad.com

Bach Flower Remedies for Emotional Support

Developed by Dr. Edward Bach in the 1930s, Bach Flower Remedies are a gentle, natural system of healing that targets emotional imbalances. Each of the 38 flower remedies is designed to address a specific emotion, such as fear, uncertainty or overwhelm, helping to restore emotional harmony. Suggested remedies are included in the Navigating Life's Challenges chapter, offering practical support for managing common emotional states.

Website: https://www.bachremedies.com

Strengths Profile – Free Starter Profile

This free tool helps you explore your unique strengths by categorising them into realised strengths, unrealised strengths, learned behaviours and weaknesses. It offers insight into how you naturally thrive and where you might focus your energy for greater fulfilment. Ideal for anyone seeking deeper self-awareness and purpose-aligned growth.

Website: https://www.strengthsprofile.com/en-us/products/free

16 Personalities – Myers-Briggs-Inspired Personality Assessment

This popular, research-based personality test provides a detailed overview of your type across four dimensions, inspired by the Myers-Briggs framework. It explores strengths, challenges, communication styles and personal growth tips. A valuable tool for understanding yourself and others better, at work, in relationships and in life.

Website: https://www.16personalities.com

Chloë Bisson – Just Write the Damn Book

A no-nonsense, motivating resource for anyone who feels they have a book inside them but doesn't know where to start. This guide helped us stay focused and finish what we started – it might just do the same for you.

Website: https://www.chloebisson.com

References

These are the studies and sources we've directly referred to throughout the book. Each chapter has its own set of references, and the superscript numbers in the text will guide you here if you'd like to learn more.

Chapter 1: Our Perception of Ageing

[1] B. R. Levy, M. D. Slade, S. R. Kunkel, and S. V. Kasl, 'Longevity Increased by Positive Self-Perceptions of Aging,' *Journal of Personality and Social Psychology*, vol. 83, no. 2, 2002, pp. 261–270.

[2] E.J. Langer., "Mindfulness and the Aging Process: A Case Study," *Journal of Personality and Social Psychology*, 57.6 (1989), 950–964..

[3] *The Young Ones* [documentary], Dir. F. Pitcher, BBC One, first broadcast 11 October 2010, https://www.bbc.co.uk/programmes/b00tq4d3.

Chapter 2: Mind-Body Connection

[1] B.H. Lipton, *The Biology of Belief: Unleashing the Power of Consciousness, Matter and Miracles*, Carlsbad, Hay House, 2005.

REFERENCES

[2] D. Chopra, *Quantum Healing: Exploring the Frontiers of Mind/Body Medicine*, New York, Bantam Books, 1989.

[3] J. Dispenza, *Becoming Supernatural: How Common People Are Doing the Uncommon*, Carlsbad, Hay House, 2017.

[4] S. Peters, *The Chimp Paradox: The Mind Management Programme to Help You Achieve Success, Confidence and Happiness*, London, Vermilion, 2012.

[5] P. Stapleton, D. Church and H. Sheldon, "A Randomised Clinical Trial of Emotional Freedom Techniques (EFT) for Psychological and Physiological Symptoms of Stress: Is EFT Effective for Reducing Stress and Anxiety?," *Journal of Nervous and Mental Disease*, 200.10 (2012), 891–896.

[6] P. Stapleton, D. Church and A. Yang, "Is Tapping on Acupuncture Points an Active Ingredient in Emotional Freedom Techniques? A Randomized Controlled Dismantling Study," *Energy Psychology: Theory, Research, and Treatment*, 5.1 (2013), 13–26.

[7] C.B. Pert, *Molecules of Emotion: The Science Behind Mind-Body Medicine*, New York, Scribner, 1997.

[8] S.W. Porges, *The Polyvagal Theory: Neurophysiological Foundations of Emotions, Attachment, Communication, and Self-Regulation*, New York: W. W. Norton, 2011.

[9] S. Roberts, *Get Strong, Get Fit, Get Happy: A Life Manual for 40+*, London, Hashtag Press, 2020.

[10] D. Chopra, *Magical Mind, Magical Body: Mastering the Mind/Body Connection for Perfect Health and Total Well-Being*, Audio CD, Nightingale-Conant, 1994.

Chapter 3: Life Wisdom

[1] R. Waldinger and M. Schulz, *The Good Life: Lessons from the World's Longest Scientific Study of Happiness*, London: Penguin Life, 2023.

[2] K. Pillemer, *30 Lessons for Living: Tried and True Advice from the Wisest Americans*, New York, Hudson Street Press, 2011.

[3] C. Wrosch, I. Bauer and M. Scheier, "Regret and Quality of Life Across the Adult Life Span: The Influence of Disengagement and Available Future Goals," *Psychology and Aging*, 20.4 (2005), 657–670.

[4] C. Wrosch and J. Heckhausen, "Perceived Control of Life Regrets: Good for Young and Bad for Old Adults," *Psychology and Aging*, 17.3 (2002), 319–330.

[5] B. Ware, *The Top Five Regrets of the Dying: A Life Transformed by the Dearly Departing*, Carlsbad, CA: Hay House, 2011.

[6] T. Robbins, *Awaken the Giant Within: How to Take Immediate Control of Your Mental, Emotional, Physical and Financial Destiny!*, New York, Simon & Schuster, 1991.

Chapter 4: Know Thyself

[1] T. Zhong, "Physical Activity Motivations and Psychological Well-Being Among University Students: A Canonical

REFERENCES

Correlation Analysis," *Frontiers in Public Health*, 12 (2024): Article 1442632. https://www.frontiersin.org/articles/10.3389/fpubh.2024.1442632/full.

[2] E. Seppälä, "The Power of Compassion and Importance of the Work of CCARE," *Center for Compassion and Altruism Research and Education*, Stanford University. https://ccare.stanford.edu/videos/power-of-compassion-importance-of-the-work-of-ccare/.

[3] P. Kaliman, M. J. Alvarez-López, M. Cosín-Tomás, *et al.*, "Rapid Changes in Histone Deacetylases and Inflammatory Gene Expression in Expert Meditators," *Psychoneuroendocrinology*, 40 (2014), 96–107. https://doi.org/10.1016/j.psyneuen.2013.11.004.

[4] R. Govindaraj, S. Nizamuddin, A. Sharath, *et al.*, "Genome-Wide Analysis Correlates Ayurveda Prakriti," *Scientific Reports*, 5 (2015): Article 15786. https://www.nature.com/articles/srep15786.

Chapter 6: Purpose and Passion

[1] P. L., Hill and N. A. Turiano, "Purpose in Life as a Predictor of Mortality Across Adulthood," *Psychological Science*, 25.7 (2014), 1482–1486. https://doi.org/10.1177/0956797614531799.

[2] C.D. Ryff, "Psychological Well-being Revisited: Advances in the Science and Practice of Eudaimonia," *Psychotherapy and Psychosomatics*, 83.1 (2014), 10–28. https://doi.org/10.1159/000353263.

[3] A. Alimujiang, A. Wiensch, J. Boss, *et al.*, "Association Between Life Purpose and Mortality Among US Adults Older Than 50

Years," *JAMA Network Open*, 2.5 (2019), e194270. https://doi.org/10.1001/jamanetworkopen.2019.4270.

[4] Harvard University, "Over Nearly 80 Years, Harvard Study Has Been Showing How to Live a Healthy and Happy Life," *Harvard Gazette*, 11 April 2017. https://news.harvard.edu/gazette/story/2017/04/over-nearly-80-years-harvard-study-has-been-showing-how-to-live-a-healthy-and-happy-life/.

[5] BetterUp, "How Motivation Works in the Brain: Exploring the Science," *BetterUp Blog*, 24 August 2022. https://www.betterup.com/blog/how-motivation-works-in-the-brain.

[6] D.C. Willcox, B.J. Willcox, W.i Hsueh, and M. Suzuki, "Okinawa Centenarian Study," *Wikipedia*, 2 January 2024. https://en.wikipedia.org/wiki/Okinawa_Centenarian_Study.

Chapter 7: Nothing Is Learned Until It Is Lived

[1] J.M.J. Murre and J. Dros, "Replication and Analysis of Ebbinghaus' Forgetting Curve," *PLOS ONE*, 10.7 (2015), e0120644. https://doi.org/10.1371/journal.pone.0120644 (accessed 10 May 2025).

[2] B.R. Levy, M.D. Slade, S.R. Kunkel, and S.V. Kasl, "Longevity Increased by Positive Self-Perceptions of Aging," *Journal of Personality and Social Psychology*, 83.2 (2002), 261–270.

[3] B.R. Levy, J.M. Hausdorff, R. Hencke and J.Y. Wei, "Reducing Age Stereotype's Influence on Physical Function: The Role of Positive Self-Perceptions of Aging," *The Journals of Gerontology: Series B*, 55.4 (2000), P205–P213.

REFERENCES

[4] K.M. Sheldon, and L.S. Krieger, "Understanding the Negative Effects of Legal Education on Law Students: A Longitudinal Test of Self-Determination Theory," *Frontiers in Psychology*, 5 (2014), 1–9

[5] Harvard T.H. Chan School of Public Health, "Social Connection Is a Major Factor in Longevity and Public Health," *Harvard T.H. Chan School of Public Health News*, 2023 https://www.hsph.harvard.edu/news/hsph-in-the-news/social-connection-longevity/ [accessed 18 July 2025]

[6] *Harvard Health Publishing*, "A Positive Mindset Can Help Your Heart," 14 February 2019. Available at: https://www.health.harvard.edu/blog/a-positive-mindset-can-help-your-heart-2019021415999 (accessed 10 May 2025).

Chapter 8: Sense of Wonder

[1] V.E. Sturm, S. Datta, A.R. Roy, et al., "Awe Walks Promote Emotional Well-Being in Older Adults," *Emotion*, 21.7 (2021), 1461–1470. https://doi.org/10.1037/emo0000876.

[2] J.E. Stellar, N. John-Henderson, C. L. Anderson, et al., "Positive Affect and Markers of Inflammation: Discrete Positive Emotions Predict Lower Levels of Inflammatory Cytokines," *Emotion*, 15.2 (2015), 129–133. https://doi.org/10.1037/emo0000033.

[3] D.R. Hawkins, *Power vs. Force: The Hidden Determinants of Human Behavior*, Carlsbad, CA, Hay House, 2014.

Bibliography

This is a collection of books and articles that helped shape our thinking and inspired many of the ideas in this book. While we may not have quoted from them directly, they've provided great insights, and we recommend them for your further exploration.

Bach, Edward. *Heal Thyself: An Explanation of the Real Cause and Cure of Disease.* London: C. W. Daniel, 1931.

Bacci, Ingrid. *The Art of Effortless Living.* London: Hodder & Stoughton, 2002.

Bronowski, J. *The Ascent of Man.* Repr. of 1973 edn. London: BBC Publications, 1979.

Burkeman, Oliver. *Meditations for Mortals: Four Weeks to Embrace Your Limitations and Make Time for What Counts.* London: The Bodley Head, 2024.

Chopra, Deepak. *Ageless Body, Timeless Mind: The Quantum Alternative to Growing Old.* London: Rider, 2008.

BIBLIOGRAPHY

Chopra, Deepak. *Reinventing the Body, Resurrecting the Soul: How to Create a New You.* London: Rider, 2009.

Chopra, Deepak. *The Book of Secrets: Unlocking the Hidden Dimensions of Your Life.* London: Rider, 2004.

Clear, James. *Atomic Habits: An Easy and Proven Way to Build Good Habits and Break Bad Ones.* London: Random House Business, 2018.

Hawkins, David R. *Power vs. Force: The Hidden Determinants of Human Behavior.* Carlsbad, CA: Hay House, 2014.

Hay, Louise. *You Can Heal Your Life.* London: Hay House, 1984.

Lipton, Bruce H. *The Biology of Belief: Unleashing the Power of Consciousness, Matter and Miracles.* Carlsbad, CA: Hay House, 2015.

McGarey, Gladys. *The Well-Lived Life: A 102-Year-Old Doctor's Six Secrets to Health and Happiness at Every Age.* London: Rider, 2023.

McLaren, Karla. *The Language of Emotions: What Your Feelings Are Trying to Tell You.* Boulder, CO: Sounds True, 2010.

Northrup, Christiane. *Goddesses Don't Age: The Secret Prescription for Radiance, Vitality, and Well-Being.* Carlsbad, CA: Hay House, 2015.

Pert, Candace B. *Molecules of Emotion: The Science Behind Mind-Body Medicine*. New York: Scribner, 1997.

Roberts, Stuart. *Get Strong, Get Fit, Get Happy*. London: Hashtag Press, 2020

Sagan, Carl. *Cosmos*. New York: Random House, 1980.

Sage, Peter. *The Inside Track: An Inspirational Guide to Conquering Adversity*. Peter Sage Publishing, 2018.

Sandberg, Sheryl, and Adam Grant. *Option B: Facing Adversity, Building Resilience, and Finding Joy*. London: WH Allen, 2017.

Sinclair, David A. *Lifespan: Why We Age – and Why We Don't Have To*. London: Thorsons, 2019.

Smith, Hyrum W. *What Matters Most: The Power of Living Your Values*. New York: Simon & Schuster, 2001.

Suzuki, Shunryu. *Zen Mind, Beginner's Mind: Informal Talks on Zen Meditation and Practice*. Boston: Shambhala Publications, 2006.

Thomson, Peter. *The Pinnacle Principle: The 5 Step Formula for Creating Extraordinary Results in Life, Business and Relationships*. Peter Thomson International, 2013.

www.ingramcontent.com/pod-product-compliance
Lightning Source LLC
Chambersburg PA
CBHW052021070526
44584CB00016B/1842